Handbook of

Medical Office Communications

Effective Letters, Memos, and E-mails

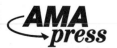

Kay Stanley, CMPE
The Coker Group

AMA Press
Vice President, Business Products: Anthony J. Frankos
Publisher: Michael Desposito
Director, Production and Manufacturing: Jean Roberts
Senior Acquisitions Editor: Marsha Mildred
Developmental Editor: Carol Brockman
Contributing Editor: Pat Dragisic
Director, Marketing: J. D. Kinney
Marketing Manager: Elizabeth Kerr
Senior Production Coordinator: Boon Ai Tan
Senior Print Coordinator: Ronnie Summers

Handbook of Medical Office Communications: Effective Letters, Memos, and E-mails

Internet address: www.ama-assn.org

Additional copies of this book may be ordered by calling 800 621-8335.
Secure online orders can be taken at www.amapress.com.
Mention product number OP142505.

ISBN 1-57947-629-5
BQ13:04-P-018:12/04

Library of Congress Cataloging-in-Publication Data

Stanley, Kay, 1944-
  Handbook of medical office communications : effective letters, memos, and e-mails / Kay Stanley.
     p. ; cm.
  Includes bibliographical references and index.
  ISBN 1-57947-629-5
  1. Communication in medicine—Handbooks, manuals, etc. 2. Medical offices—Handbooks, manuals, etc.
  [DNLM: 1. Correspondence—Handbooks. 2. Professional Practice—Handbooks. 3. Electronic Mail—Handbooks. 4. Interprofessional Relations—Handbooks. 5. Professional-Patient Relations—Handbooks. W 49 S788h 2005] I. Title.

R118.S775 2005
  808'.06661—dc22   2004017615

CONTENTS

Too much of today's business writing is needlessly difficult to understand or, worse, conveys the wrong message. Nonverbal mediums, such as e-mail, faxes, letters, memos, and instruction sheets, that are intended to give direction are frequently misused or written poorly, causing misunderstandings and incorrect assumptions. Medical practices are particularly vulnerable when patients are unable to comprehend the message, whatever the medium used. And employees are frequently confused and often demoralized by communications received from management, particularly when the communication is one-way (nonverbal) and not in the context of a conversation. Privacy is an extremely important issue for transferring patient information, and, when communication is not handled correctly, it can expose the practice to unnecessary liability and risk.

Handbook of Medical Office Communications: Effective Letters, Memos, and E-mails provides readers a handy resource for achieving a level of excellence for both external (patient-related) and internal (employee-related) communications. Remembering that the physician's practice is a busy place with many people coming and going about their work, the intent is to simplify the written communications process by setting up logical standards and providing easy-to-use samples. Most people do not like to write, but even those who do could brush up on ways to capture their reader's attention, encourage action, promote goodwill, and get results.

Each chapter will elaborate on the reasons for writing and composing in a certain way and within established parameters to accomplish your goals as the writer. You will discover ways to compose letters and memos faster by following proven techniques for planning, organizing, formatting, writing, and editing the most frequently used documents in the medical practice. Samples of letters and memos will include hints for an ideal letter as well as analyses of poor letters so that you can understand why some words, phrases, tones, and tenses should and should not be included in written communications. The CD-ROM that accompanies this book also provides working files (in Microsoft Word format) of letters featured throughout this book. Consider using these files as templates and adapting them to create your organization's correspondences. Additionally, the appearance of a communication says much about an organization's professionalism.

The underlying theme of this book is the significant role—negative and positive—that written communication plays in both patient satisfaction and compliance and employee satisfaction and compliance. The goal will be to achieve a positive effect and enhance your credibility with each communiqué.

ABOUT THE AUTHOR

Kay Stanley, CMPE, joined The Coker Group, a national health care consulting firm in Atlanta, Georgia, in 1988 and currently serves as associate partner. Heading the company's publishing and education initiative, Ms Stanley's responsibilities involve development, production, and sales of Coker's books, manuals, and the monthly newsletter *CokerConnection*. Works directly credited to Ms Stanley include *OSHA Hazard Communications, A Guide for Dermatology Practices; Bloodborne Pathogens, A Guide for Dermatology Practices;* and *Personnel Management in the Medical Practice, Second Edition* (AMA Press). Articles attributed to Ms Stanley are published in *Practice Pointers* (American Osteopathic Association) and *Urology Times*.

Ms Stanley has more than 20 years of experience in administration, personnel, and editorial management. She is a member of the Medical Group Management Association at the local, state, and national levels, and she speaks at workshops on current issues. Ms Stanley is a Certified Medical Practice Executive of the American College of Medical Practice Executives. She also serves on the Educational Advisory Council for the American Medical Association's KnowledgeLink® Educational Programs. A member of the Healthcare Financial Management Association, Ms Stanley serves as coeditor of the *Georgia Scroll*.

The Coker Group, a leader in health care consulting, helps providers improve financial and operational results through sound business principles. The consulting team members are proficient, trustworthy professionals with experience and strengths in various areas. The well-rounded staff includes seasoned individuals in finance, administration, management, operations, compliance, personnel management, and information systems.

The Coker Group's nationwide client base includes major health systems, hospitals, physician groups, and solo practitioners in a full spectrum of engagements. The Coker Group has gained a reputation since 1987 for thorough, efficient, and cost-conscious work to benefit its clients financially and operationally. The firm has a towering profile with recognized and respected health care professionals throughout the industry. Coker's exceptional consulting team has health care, technical, financial, and business knowledge and offers comprehensive programs, services, and training to yield long-term solutions and turnarounds. Coker staff members are devoted to delivering reliable answers and dependable options so that decision makers can make categorical decisions. Coker consultants enable providers to concentrate on patient care.

Service Areas

- Practice management, billing and collection reviews, chart audits
- Procedural coding analysis
- Information systems review, including electronic medical records
- Physician employment and compensation review
- Physician network development
- Practice appraisals
- Strategic/business planning
- Disengagements of practices and network unwinds
- Practice operational assessments
- Contract negotiations
- Hospital services, medical staff development
- Practice startups
- Buy/sell and equity analysis
- Sale/acquisition negotiations
- Group formation and dissolution
- Educational programs, workshops, and training
- Compliance plans

- Health Insurance Portability and Accountability Act assessments and compliance
- Management services organization (MSO) development
- Financial analysis
- Mediation and expert witnessing
- Policies and procedures manuals

For more information, contact:

The Coker Group
11660 Alpharetta Hwy, Suite 710
Roswell, GA 30076
800 345-5829
www.cokergroup.com

The Importance of a Well-Written Communication

For the right reasons, people will make numerous sacrifices for an organization or a community. But they need to be reminded of their nobility and thanked for it. The same holds true for your patients and your staff.

As a physician, your patients and staff need something to make them trust your leadership. People put their trust in other people—not plans or blueprints or five-year strategies or projections. It's the relationship that matters. Delivering your message in a way your audience appreciates (even if they don't necessary like its meaning) is fundamental to political success.

None of this means that context is everything and content is nothing. For some audiences the analytical, black-and-white message may be exactly the right tone and approach for success.

It also doesn't mean that every message you deliver should be touchy-feely, let's-hold-hands moments. It's almost always a mix of heart and head.

It means you must think about your audience before you think about your message. It means you must position what you say in terms that are not just clear, but meaningful to them. It means you and your team must have active relationships with every group of constituents that can help or hurt your organization.

> "It's not what you tell your players that counts—it's what they hear."
>
> Red Auerbach,
> Coach of the Boston Celtics[1]

The language barrier is yours to build or crush. The purpose of this chapter is to see the relationship between good written communication, patient and employee satisfaction, and the success of your practice.

PATIENT RELATIONS AND SATISFACTION

Health care providers are prone to think that competition is about quality, but quality is hard to measure, and to some degree patient satisfaction is a measure of perceived quality. Nevertheless, patient satisfaction will be the final differentiator between medical practices that are successful and those that flounder or fail. Why? Because health care consumers have more choices today than they've had in the past and they are less hesitant to move from one physician to another.

For this reason, total patient satisfaction is the number one goal of every successful organization. Understand that the pursuit of health care is a highly intense process for your patients. Your practice can have the most highly trained and efficient staff and procedures, but if patients are not well informed, their perception is likely to be poor. Patients' anxiousness is usually relieved with frequent communication about the status of their case.

The type of communication is just as important as the frequency of communication. A standardized content for messages—verbal or written—should be learned by all staff. Each message would include the following components:

- A kind, caring attitude
- A willingness to provide more information and explanation if called for
- Updates and feedback on what to expect
- Reassurance that it is of personal importance the patient be cared for quickly

Take a look at what measures you are using to send "patient satisfaction" messages to your patients. When patients know that you are concerned about their perception, they are more inclined to regard your practice with graciousness. Further, more communication from the top of the organization, more frequently, and via more channels makes the message have an impact on the staff. Begin your patient satisfaction communication initiative through a written pledge stating your philosophy of respect (see Figure 1-1). Your patient satisfaction pledge should be printed on your practice brochure and on framed copies throughout your facility.

View your communications from the patient's perspective and determine how you would receive that information from another professional. Did you project a kind and caring attitude? Did you offer to provide more information if the patient feels confused or wants to know more?

FIGURE 1-1

Patient Satisfaction Pledge

Welcome to Hope Medical Clinic, where you are more than a patient or visitor. You are our guest. We are dedicated to serving you with dignity, kindness, and courtesy. Your satisfaction is our primary concern. We appreciate the opportunity to be of service to you.

                                        Physician's (or Chief Executive Officer's) Name

Have you followed up on what you have promised to deliver in the way of feedback or further education? Have you considered the patient's level of anxiety and desire to have immediate attention? Have you examined your tone and did you mean to sound like that? Did you say what you meant to say? Finally, did you let the patient know the reason and what to expect?

Correlation of Patient Education to Patient Satisfaction

A patient's expectations and perception of a service are integral to his or her satisfaction levels. The closer the experience resembles expectations, the more satisfied the patient will be. Therefore, early education on what to expect in each step or stage of the process shapes the patient's expectations to be closer to reality. The more closely the experience resembles expectations, the more satisfied the patient will be.

To the extent that most clinical outcomes rely on how well patients follow physicians' posttreatment instructions, patient education again plays a dominant role in overall satisfaction. When patients understand why certain behaviors are prescribed and required and the ramifications if protocols are not followed, they are more likely to follow through on instructions and therefore to have better outcomes.

Obtaining Communication on Patient Satisfaction

Communication is a two-way street by its very nature; there is a sender and a receiver. You can establish healthy dialogue with your patients in written form through comment cards. By collecting feedback from patients and visitors, you will gain valuable insight about your practice and set in motion an expectation of positive communication—even if the information you receive is negative. The "We Care Card," in Figure 1-2, will allow you to learn what you are doing well and therefore should be doing more of, and it tells you where improvements are needed, and perhaps even how to make the improvements.

Ask your patients what they want. They will tell you. Then do a good job providing it. If you do this across the board, little by little you will start to transform the organization. No longer will you be like every other medical practice. You will, in marketing terms, differentiate yourself.

One of the first ways you want to differentiate yourself is in courtesy and respect by making your practice warm and friendly. Then ask your patients for a list of all the other things that you may not even have thought about.

A welcome letter is another way to express your practice philosophy of patient satisfaction and to develop an enduring relationship with your patients. Be sure that your message contains the essential components of caring, willingness to explain, prompt and accurate feedback, and reassurance of the importance of each individual. Figure 1-3 offers a model welcome letter.

FIGURE 1-2

We Care Card

Hope Medical Clinic is dedicated to listening and responding to your needs. At Hope Medical Clinic, we are interested in your comments, concerns, and compliments. Please complete this form and return it at the drop box in the reception area. Or simply detach this postage-paid card and drop into any US mailbox.

Comments: _____

_____

Complaints: _____

_____

_____

Compliments: _____

_____

OPTIONAL

Name: _____

Address: _____

City: _____ State: _____ Zip: _____

Phone: _____

Date response received: _____

Date forwarded to manager: _____

Date action taken: _____

EMPLOYEE RELATIONS AND SATISFACTION

Patient satisfaction can be achieved only when there is satisfaction at every level in the organization. You cannot maintain a level of patient satisfaction without a staff that is also satisfied with their working environment and wants to see your practice succeed. Because busy medical practices routinely operate in a crisis management mode with more demands on people than is reasonable, communication must be frequent and clear and channels of communication varied to gain and retain your staff's attention.

Verbal and written communications must look like the following:

- Address the most recent feedback on patient satisfaction
- Identify top irritations or issues
- Establish problem-solving groups around the top issues
- Determine the status of solutions to previous unresolved problems
- Devise additional ideas for improving patient satisfaction

FIGURE 1-3

Sample Welcome Letter

[Physician's Letterhead]

[Date]

Dear _____,

Welcome to Hope Medical Clinic. I want to give you my personal commitment that our doctors and staff will do everything possible to exceed your expectations for quality medical care, comfort, and peace of mind. We are dedicated to listening and responding to your needs.

Our office hours are Monday through Thursday from 9:00 a.m. to 5:00 p.m. Friday office hours are 9:00 a.m. to 12:00 p.m. (noon). After hours, our physicians are available for emergencies. You may contact our main line and dial "zero," which will connect you directly to our answering service, who will notify the physician who is on call.

Please use our telephone messaging center to guide you through the appropriate steps to meet your needs. Our telephone lines are always available to leave messages for prescriptions and other questions. Our staff will make every effort to respond to your call or act upon your request within a 24-hour timeframe.

Thank you in advance for giving Hope Medical Clinic an opportunity to help you enjoy better health.

Sincerely,

Gordon Goodman, MD

How do these factors relate to the importance of well-written communication? The answer is that your staff deserves and requires the same caring attitude and respect for their concerns as your patients. Every internal policy, memorandum, e-mail, and written note that you write has a tone that communicates information that will either endear you to the people who work for and with you or drive a wedge in your employee relations.

On the other hand, every communication is an opportunity for you to encourage, educate, inform, and direct your staff to achieve both patient and employee satisfaction with your practice. So the objective is to convey a kind, caring attitude, a willingness to provide more information and explanation if called for, updates and feedback on what to expect, and reassurance that the employee is of personal importance to the practice.

CONCLUSION

What the patient really wants is what the patient wants. If you give your patients what they want, they will be satisfied. If you give them more than they expect, they will be ecstatic. All patients and physicians are individuals with unique quirks and idiosyncrasies, specific opinions they are predisposed to hold (some of which are formidable), and specific requests that will make their encounter with you more pleasant for them. If the goal is to create health care experiences that exceed patients' expectations and satisfy patients' needs at a memorable level, the health care experience must be somewhat customized for each patient.

One way to achieve that end is to be able to write well-written communiqués to your patients, based on attention to patients' personal concerns, respect for the patients' health problems, and content and phrasing that leaves little to misunderstand yet opens the door for follow-up and pursuit of more information, if necessary. When your communications are well planned and well written, your practice will experience great rewards over the long term.

ENDNOTE

1. Maxwell JC. Playing over their heads. *Leadership Wired.* February 2004;7, no. 4. Available at: http://www.injoy.com/leadershipwired/. Accessed March 18, 2004.

chapter 2

The Letter and Memo Writing Process

Most medical practices are so busy with many activities and tasks that the importance of communicating well through the written word may be underestimated. On the other hand, others tasked with drafting communiqués—whether informed consent forms, patient bills, educational handouts, memorandums, or correspondence—may be so concerned about their impact that they are reticent to put anything in writing. Composing your practice's documents is time consuming and burdensome for most people. The average person, in fact, may find it difficult to get started in drafting written work. The purpose of this chapter is to lay out the three stages of letter and memo writing:

1. Prewriting (preparation)
2. Writing (composition)
3. Editing (or revising)

Whether you are writing to your patients, your staff, or an institution (eg, an insurance company, hospital, or organization), you can save time, reduce your stress, and make your correspondence more reader-oriented if you follow each stage.

Remember the goal: to communicate to the reader the message that you intend to convey. Most often, this is best accomplished through plain-style English.

PREPARATION

A well-planned letter or memo depends on clear thinking before you ever write your first sentence. By planning and organizing, you can reduce needless first, second, or third attempts at writing. So, before you start, consider these questions:

- Is the letter or memo necessary?
- Can you make a telephone call or send a form letter instead?
- What is your purpose? What do you want this document to accomplish? Is it to inform your reader? Is it to ask for information or

action? Is it to persuade? Is it to propose an idea? Is it to create a good impression?

- Who is your reader? Consider age, gender, position, education, knowledge of subject, personality style, interest level, biases, and reaction to your subject. Is this follow-up correspondence? What does your reader want or need? When? Why? How much does your reader already know? How can you help your reader? Do you expect a reply?

- What are the key points to cover? Think about your purpose, visualize your reader, and think through your ideas. Jot down a word or two on each key point that needs covering. Go back later and put them in the best order.

- What do you want your reader to do? What response or action do you expect? For example, do you want your reader to read your letter and file it? Read it and toss it? Read it and take action? Read it and pass it on to another reader? If you want your reader to call you, do you say, "Please call me by 3:00 on Friday," or do you say, "Please contact me this week"? Figure 2-1 gives an example of stating what you want the reader to do.

Be sure to state the specific response or action you want from your reader at the end of your letter or memo.

Overcoming Writer's Block

If you have ever tried to start a letter and nothing comes to mind, you are experiencing what is known as writer's block. You can use any of these techniques to get off to a good start.

- Talk it out. Imagine yourself talking to your reader, and write what you would say in your conversation. You will go back later and revise what you have said.

F I G U R E   2 - 1

Defining a Response

Dear Mr. Smith:

So that you can maintain your credit with us, please send your payment of $125.00 by November 30, 2004. We want to continue working with you and providing you with the patient care you have come to expect from us.

Thank you for making the payment.

Sincerely,
Northside Medical Group

"I don't know where to begin," said Alice.

"Begin at the beginning," suggested Humpty-Dumpty, "Go on until you come to the end, and then stop."

—from *Through the Looking Glass*

- Listing. List the ideas that you want to include and put them in the order that you will cover them. Then turn the ideas into complete thoughts.

- Outlining. Some writers like to use outlining (see Figure 2-2).

- Five Ws and one H. Answer each of these questions: who, what, where, when, why, and how. The answers will convey the most important ideas.

- Clustering or mind mapping. Draw a circle in the center of your page. Write the purpose of your letter or memo in the circle. Then generate your main ideas and lace them in small circles connected by straight lines to your main circle. As you create subsidiary ideas to the main ideas, you can show those in even smaller circles that are connected by straight lines to the second tier of circles. Once you finish creating your ideas, put them in a logical order (see Figure 2-3).

COMPOSITION

After you plan and organize your ideas, you will turn them into sentences and paragraphs. In this stage, you will write a rough draft—not a perfect piece—without concern for grammar, punctuation, spelling, usage, capitalization, or word choice. Composing is more important than cleanup—correcting can occur in the editing stage.

Bear in mind your audience and your patient demographics. "Literacy researchers recommend writing at a junior-high reading level. However, studies show people often read three to five grades lower than their highest level of educational attainment, so someone with a high school diploma may actually read at a seventh- to ninth-grade level."[1]

FIGURE 2-2

Using an Outline

I. Announcement of new office location

  A. New address

    1. Why we are moving

      a. Need larger space

      b. Need to be closer to patients

    2. Directions to office

  B. Benefits to patients

    1. Accessible to public transportation

    2. Easier to find

    3. Newer facility

II. Gracious and sincere close

F I G U R E   2 - 3

Mind Mapping Your Thoughts

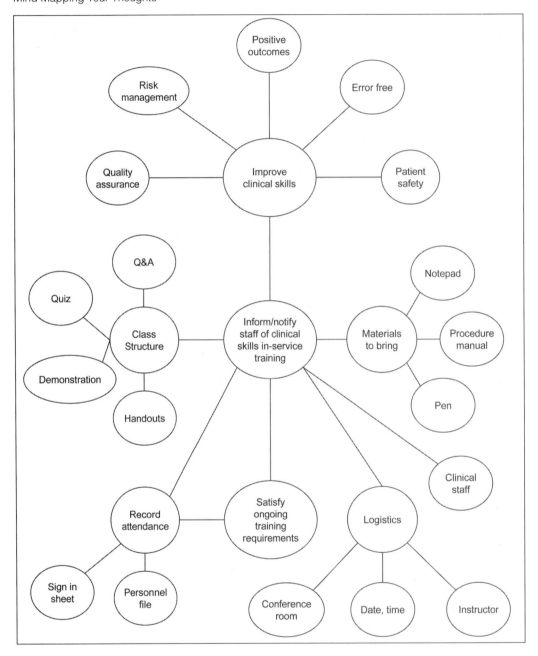

Use plain language. Do not worry about appearing to be too elementary in your documents. You are unlikely to ever hear a patient complain that your written materials are too simple to understand.

Once you have your content, you will go over the text ruthlessly to eliminate any confusing phraseology.

Appearance and form are important, too, but will be covered in another section.

EDITING

Editing is the time to review your rough draft and polish it. Read it and check for organization, sentence structure, spelling, usage, grammar, punctuation, and capitalization. This is the time to check your content for facts, dates, and amounts, and other details that must be accurate, particularly in the patient-physician relationship. Eliminate medical jargon and archaic words and phrases that will be hard for your reader to understand.

An error commonly made is to use unnecessary words, which weakens your message and leaves room for confusion. On the other hand, avoid using contractions (which is the elimination of parts of words). Seldom are contractions considered professional in formal correspondence, and they can be easily misunderstood when read hastily. The checklist provided in Table 2-1 will help you in editing your composition.

Finally, take a break and then go back to your writing. If you read it aloud, you will be more aware of whether your sentences are too long, subjects and verbs agree, your choice of tense is appropriate, etc. Have another person review your letter or memo. Read it again, pretending that you are the reader. Recheck your facts, statistics, dates, and amounts for accuracy. Check the basics for smooth transition, verbs, jargon, wordiness, and visual layout. Be ruthless as you critique your own writing.

In the section that follows, you will learn more about ways to edit your work.

T A B L E   2 - 1

Reviewer's Checklist for the Writing Process

❑ Have you eliminated unnecessary words and phrases?

❑ Are dates, numbers, names, and facts accurate?

❑ Are sentences complete?

❑ Do subjects and verbs agree?

❑ Have archaic words, professional jargon, and redundancies been removed?

❑ Have you stated the purpose at the beginning?

❑ Is the letter or memo reader friendly?

❑ Have you clearly stated the desired action?

❑ Do your sentences flow logically and smoothly?

❑ Have you answered your reader's questions?

❑ Have you used active voice more than passive voice?

❑ Is the writing conversational?

❑ Have you used the appropriate tone?

❑ Have you used contractions?

Strengthening Your Writing Style: When Less Is Better

Lewis Carroll's whimsical tale of a conversation between Humpty Dumpty and Alice cleverly conveys the problem of miscommunication and the ensuing annoyance. When physicians talk to their patients by using words or terminology that the patients don't understand, they can expect patients to be annoyed, at a minimum. More serious is the problem of lack of compliance.

> "When I use a word, it means just what I choose it to mean—neither more nor less."
>
> Humpty Dumpty
> —from *Through the Looking Glass*

Medical practices spend considerable time and resources developing materials about specific health issues, treatment options, and step-by-step instructions to educate patients about how they can aid in their own recovery. Unfortunately, patients often don't understand these materials, partly because they are generally written at an eighth- to 11th-grade reading level, while 90 million Americans either are functionally illiterate or have reading skills at or below the fifth-grade reading level. The reality is that patients with low literacy skills have significant problems understanding and effectively using the health care information available to them.[2]

It is for this reason that you must make every effort to achieve clarity and conciseness and convey the right tone throughout every mode of communication that occurs in your medical practice. You can strengthen your communication with your patients by strengthening your style in the following ways.

- **Use short, simple words.** A major cause of wordy, unclear writing is the use of inflated words instead of simple ones. Inflated words may have the same meaning, but they clutter your writing, confuse your reader, and make your writing sound phony and stilted. Minimize problems of misunderstanding by using common words, defining uncommon words, and giving examples that show readers how to connect health information to their lives.

Inflated Words	Simple Words
Procure	Get
Endeavor	Try
Utilization	Use
Disseminate	Spread
Substantiate	Support
Administer	Give

- **Eliminate wordy expressions.** Beware of needless phrases often introduced by prepositions like at, on, for, in, to, and by. They weaken your writing by cluttering the meaning. Instead be natural and friendly.

Wordy	Simple
Due to the fact that	Because
In order to	To
In the amount of $50	For $50
In the city of Atlanta	In Atlanta
By means of	By
At the present time	Now
Prior to the start of	Before

■ **Remove redundancies.** Redundancies—words that say the same thing twice—are a sign of careless thinking. Examples:

Redundant	Simple
Refer back	Refer
Fill out and complete	Complete
Definite decision	Decision
Plan ahead	Plan
Very unique	Unique
Advance warning	Warning
Qualified expert	Expert
Still remains	Remains
Totally destroyed	Destroyed
Postpone until later	Postpone
Merge together	Merge
Personal opinion	Opinion

■ **Avoid clichés.** Recognize and remove trite and archaic expressions, which often lurk in beginnings and endings. Instead, use crisp and original language.

Outdated	Updated
Enclosed please find	Enclosed is
Please be advised that	[omit]
This office is in receipt of your letter	Thank you for your letter
As per your request	Regarding your request
Please do not hesitate to contact	Please call
Please feel free to call	Please call
Thanking you in advance for your cooperation	Thank you for your help
Hoping to hear from you soon	I would appreciate hearing from you by (mo/day/year)

■ **Avoid archaic, technical, and legalistic jargon.** Some writers automatically slip into another mode that differs from their everyday speech patterns. Instead of writing naturally as they would speak, their use of archaic, technical, or legalistic jargon only serves to make their letters cold, impersonal, pompous, and unnatural. Keep your writing current and up to date by using a down-to-earth style. Be particularly cognizant of using the technical jargon of the medical profession and realize that your reader may not understand terms that are familiar to you. When using acronyms, spell them out the first time they are used, as in American Medical Association (AMA), and use the acronym alone afterward.

Outdated	Updated
This writer	I
Duly noted	Received, see
Find herewith	Enclosed
Kindly	Please
Pursuant to our agreement	As we agreed
Herein	Below

- **Use gender-neutral language.** Avoid offending one of the sexes by either using gender-neutral language or staying clear of sexist phrases.

Sexist	Gender Neutral
Mankind	People
To man	To staff, operate
Salesman	Sales representative
Fireman	Fire fighter

A second solution is to rewrite your sentence in the plural.

From: Each patient must pay his bill at the time of service.

To: Patients must pay their bills at the time of service.

Or address your reader in the second person.

From: The patient must complete the form before his appointment.

To: Complete your form before your appointment.

A safe bet is to avoid using pronouns whenever possible.

From: Each patient must present his insurance card at every appointment.

To: Each patient must present an insurance card at every appointment.

- **Use active verbs.** A sentence is active when the subject acts; it is passive when the subject receives the action. Generally, active verbs give life, promote action, and personalize your writing. Passive verbs, in contrast, slow down your reader, muddle your meaning, and weaken the message. The active voice gives clearer direction; the passive sentence is ambiguous and slows down the reader. Not all instances of passive voice are inappropriate, however, and some uses are necessary. The writer should be aware of being as clear as possible when communicating a message or instructions.

Active	Passive
We received your lab results today.	The results of your lab report were received today.
Bring your filled out form with you to your appointment.	Your form should be filled out before you arrive for your appointment.

Active	**Passive**
We received your employment inquiry today.	This letter will acknowledge receipt of your inquiry regarding employment opportunities.

- **Avoid "smothered verbs."** Avoid smothering verbs by watching for words that end in *-ive, -sion, -ment, -ence, -ance,* or *-tion.* Making verbs into nouns deadens your writing, bores your reader, and makes you appear indecisive, which tempts the reader to ignore or skip over what you are writing. A tipoff that you are smothering verbs is overuse of the words *make, give, take,* and *come.* The point is, write with everyday verbs.

Smothered	**Uncovered**
Your insurance company gave authorization for us to perform the procedure.	Your insurance company authorized us to perform the procedure.
Upon doing an examination of your x-rays, we have come to the conclusion that the surgery is indicated.	After examining your x-rays, we conclude that you need surgery.
Her report made the implication that the hospital failed to provide adequate safety for the patient.	Her report implied that the hospital failed to adequately protect the patient.

- **Use short sentences.** The language of business documents should be as concise as you can make it. Wordiness detracts from precision, while short sentences add strength, vitality, and clarity to your writing. A sentence should be long enough to get your message across, yet short enough to be energetic. Keep the following ideas firmly in mind:

  —**Readers expect you to come to the point.** Keep the average sentence length to 15 to 20 words or fewer.

  —**Readers expect economy of expression.** Limit each sentence to one main idea.

  —**Readers expect you to use words they understand.** Avoid medical jargon and acronyms.

  —**Readers expect you to conform to standard English.** Occasional long sentences are fine, provided they flow smoothly and are well punctuated.

- **Keep related words together.** Pick the subject and then introduce the verb early in the sentence to let the reader know what the subject is doing. Place modifiers—words, phrases, or clauses—next to the word they are meant to describe.

Misplaced	**Well Placed**
No liquids will be taken by patients having surgery after midnight.	Patients having surgery should not take liquids after midnight.

Misplaced	Well Placed
Bring your form with you that is already filled out to your appointment.	Fill out your form and bring it with you to your appointment.

■ **Be positive in your tone.** The tone of a business letter from a medical practice or communication with a patient should always be positive. Some words automatically connote positive thoughts; others are innately negative. When possible, emphasize the good news, not the bad. Soften unpleasant ideas with positive wording.

Positive	Negative
We have noticed	It is obvious
Please	You must
We ask that	You have to
Our practice is	It is our policy to
You can	You can't
You mentioned, state	You claim that

■ **Use personal pronouns.** Write as though you are talking to the patient (or to the reader, in case of a vendor or other party). Ultimately, you will want to test documents on your patients to learn what they don't understand.

The objective in this section is to demonstrate ways of writing better so that the reader connects with the meaning you intend to convey. It's not always about writing briefly. It is more about making every word count.

CONCLUSION

In this chapter, we have examined what it takes to get started in writing a good communiqué. The vehicle can be a business letter, memorandum, or policy. The same principles apply, whether the addressee is a patient, an employee, a vendor, an associate, or a peer. To strengthen your writing style, write concisely, in plain English, making every word count.

ENDNOTES

1. Hockhauser M. It's Greek to me: can your practice's documents pass the readability test? *MGMA Connexion*. January 2002:66.
2. Mayer G, Villaire M. Steps for improving health literacy. Available at: http://www.coding-compliance.com/cgi-bin/article.cgi?article_id= 1571. Accessed January 27, 2004.

The Professional Letter

Chapter 1 addressed the importance of communicating well with the patient base and with employees in the success of the medical practice for a variety of reasons. Essentially, poor or abrasive communication will hinder the level of patient satisfaction and compliance and will agitate employees as well.

Chapter 2 offered ways to construct a communiqué and to edit your work to improve your style. The objective is to communicate clearly through the use of sound composition and editing principles.

Taking nothing for granted, this chapter is devoted to the formalities and details of construction that enhance the professional image of your communications. You could say that Chapter 3 is what everyone needs to know about assembling a professional letter. The goal is to create and maintain a level of uniformity in letter writing in an effort to save time and cover all the bases of structure.

COMPONENTS

A professional letter from your medical practice will have the name of the practice and its address, the date of the correspondence, an inside address, a salutation, a body, a complimentary close, and a signature line. In addition, it will have certain options that serve useful purposes of documentation, identification, and notification. Optional parts of a letter may include a special notation, a subject line, reference initials, enclosure notation, delivery identification, copy notation, and even a postscript.

Letterhead

Every professional letter should have the name, address, telephone number, and fax number of the practice. The best way to present this information is by using standard "letterhead," which is usually printed professionally. However, through the use of computers and high-quality printers, you may be able to create your own letterhead for your practice that incorporates graphic art, such as a logo, along with the tasteful use of fonts available through your computer software. Typically, the practice name is at the top of the page, but the address can be positioned at either the top or the bottom. In Figure 3-1, the letterhead positions all the information about the practice at the top of the page. Only the first page has the name, address, telephone number, and fax number of the organization.

FIGURE 3-1

Letterhead

Hope Medical Clinic, PC

1575 Medical Center Drive, Suite 700
Birmingham, AL 25350
205.555.1200
205.555.1234 Fax

The pages that follow, or the "second sheets," typically are plain or have a logo at the bottom of the page (see Figure 3-2).

Date

Formal business letters use the unabbreviated month, day, and year, as in November 30, 2004. Informal internal memorandums and policy manuals sometimes use abbreviations or shortened forms, such as Nov. 30, 2004, 11-30-04, or 11/30/04. Military offices, governmental agencies, and many foreign countries prefer to use the date first and no punctuation, as in 30 November 2004. Place the date approximately 2 inches from the top of the page (usually line 13) or three lines below the letterhead.

Inside Address

The inside address, as a part of a professional letter, is a duplicate of the outside address and should follow the preferred format of the US Postal Service. The order is as follows:

> Addressee name
> Addressee title and department (if applicable)
> Organization name
> Street number and name
> City, State, Zip Code

Positioned on the fifth line, below the date, the inside address should be single spaced and aligned at the left margin. If you are sending the same letter to two or more people at different addresses, type the addresses one under the other (with one space between) or position them side by side. Type an envelope for each individual, omitting reference to the other recipients.

Be sure that you spell everything correctly for a couple of reasons. First, you diminish your professionalism by making errors, and second, you are apt to have an undeliverable piece of mail if you make errors in an address.

Consider using two lines for a long title or company name, as in this example of a letter to an insurance payer:

> Ms. Fredericka Vanderbilt
> Northwestern Claims Manager
> Blue Cross/Blue Shield of Massachusetts

Ordinarily, it is not applicable to use an academic degree with an inside address.

Handling the address information is extremely critical and requires much attention to detail. Items are frequently lost in the postal system if they are addressed incorrectly. Here are some fine points to consider in the address lines to increase the likelihood that your correspondence will be delivered to your intended recipient:

FIGURE 3-2

Second Sheet

Hope Medical Clinic, PC

- Spell out numbers one through ten: 11207 Seventh Street
- Type figures/numerals for street numbers higher than ten: 2004 West 42nd Street
- Do not abbreviate a compass direction if it appears before a street name (unless space is limited): 409 West Fourth Street
- Abbreviate compound direction as follows (a comma before and without a period after): 11660 Lincoln Avenue, SW
- Spell out a compass direction (if not compound) following a street name; do not use a comma: 2994 Park Avenue East
- If using a post office box number, any of the following options is permissible: PO Box 11207; Post Office Box 11207; or Box 11207.
- If your correspondence is to be delivered by a courier (eg, messenger, Federal Express, United Parcel Service, etc), you must use a street address. Post office boxes are limited to use by the United States Postal Service (USPS).

Salutation

Align the salutation at the left margin, on the third line below the inside address. Follow it with a colon as in the following example:

Dear Mr. Parson:

Only if you know the individual very well is it permissible to use the first name of the addressee, and in that case, you may use a comma after the name:

Dear Jack,

You may abbreviate titles, such as Mr., Mrs., Ms., and Dr., but you should spell out Professor, Bishop, Judge, Father, or Sister.

Referring to the reader by title (eg, Dear Customer Service Representative) is preferable to "Dear Sir" or "Gentlemen"; however, in extremely formal correspondence, you may use "Dear Sir or Madam" or "Ladies and Gentlemen."

You may also eliminate the salutation altogether by using a subject line rather than a salutation, when that is a more appropriate choice. An example of this would be a letter to a third-party payer to appeal a denial of a claim for reimbursement.

Use a reader's name whenever possible. You have the best opportunity to receive personal attention if your letter is addressed to a name of the person who should receive it. If you cannot find the name through research or other means, the next best option is to use a title. Regardless, using "To Whom It May Concern" is archaic, and its generality is even a bit offensive to some recipients.

If you do not know the gender of the addressee, use the name or initials offered rather than offend. Some names and initials are gender neutral, such as Pat, Tony, Ashley, Brook, McKenzie, and T.J. To be safe, use: Dear T.J. Murray, or Dear Pat Guise.

When addressing two people, spell out "and" instead of using an ampersand (&).

Incorrect: Dear Mr. Reynolds & Ms. Lawrence

Correct: Dear Mr. Reynolds and Ms. Lawrence

Body of the Letter

The text that contains your message begins on the second line below the salutation (or the second line below the subject line, if used). Although the length of the letter is not significant, content broken up into several brief paragraphs is favorable to longer ones.

Complimentary Closing

Place your polite ending of your letter on the second line below the last line in the body of the letter. Follow it with a comma. For professional letters, the closings most commonly used today are "Sincerely" and "Cordially."

Signature Line

Type the writer's name four lines below the complimentary closing. You may expand this space to six blank lines for very short letters or two or three lines for very long letters.

Include special title (eg, MD), relevant title, and department information, arranged on two or three lines to be visually pleasing. For example:

James Oglethorpe, MD
Medical Director
Oncology Department

If the name is gender neutral or in the case of initials, it is acceptable to use a courtesy title, such as the following:

Sincerely,
Ms. T.J. Murray
Practice Administrator

For two signatures, type signature blocks either side by side or one below the other. If side by side, place the complimentary closing aligned with the left margin, and place one signature block at the left margin, the other at the center. If using one above and one below, type the second block four lines below the end of the first block, at either the left margin or the center, depending on the format style. (Formatting will be covered in Chapter 4.)

OPTIONS

For good reasons you may choose to use reference options and notations in your professional letters. Each of the following items has significance and may be especially beneficial for correspondence generated from a medical practice. The very nature of informing patients of health care information and handling private patient information requires tracking of delivery and distribution of correspondence to patients and others.

Special Notations

Letters that are personal or confidential should be so noted directly under the date at the left margin. You may use whatever style you prefer, for example, all capitals, or initial capitals and lowercase in boldface print. Generally, use of special fonts and enhanced text functions are preferable to underscoring.

Reference notations are typed two lines below the date or two lines below any other notation that follows a date (eg, "personal" or "confidential"). Examples are as follows:

    Refer to: Policy #2681107
    Reference: Patient 8542361
    Refer to: Order #9612

Subject Line

Although the subject line is usually omitted in a physician's letter to a patient, using this notation is a useful way to replace the salutation of the letter, particularly when you are not addressing the correspondence to a specific person. A good example would be in writing to a third-party payer about a claim in question. In this case, you may not have the name of a specific person; rather, you are addressing a department, such as "Claims Department."

The subject line indicates the contents and assists in creating a frame of reference. It saves explanation time for the writer and the reader by clearly stating a purpose. An example of an appropriate use would be the following:

    SUBJECT: Request for review of denied claim

Usually typed in uppercase letters, the subject line aligns with the left margin in the extreme block style, or in the case of indented paragraphs, it is indented to align with the first line of each paragraph. When no salutation is used, a subject line is typed on the third line below the inside address. Otherwise, it is typed between the salutation and the body of the letter with one blank line above and below it.

Reference Initials

Reference initials identify the author and the typist. However, current trends are to provide the typist's initials alone when the author's name is placed in the signature block. This is particularly relevant when the author is also the typist, which occurs frequently in business and in medical practice. Using either uppercase or lowercase letters, place these initials two lines below the writer's name and title. If the writer's initials are used as well, they are always presented first, as in the following examples:

JKL/MSR
jkl:msr
JKL

Either a slash or a colon may be used.

Enclosure Notation

By typing the word "Enclosure" or an abbreviation of the word (ie, encl:, enc) at the left margin, two lines below the reference initials, you are alerting the reader that specific information has been included with the letter. As an optional clarification, you may indicate a number that represents the quantity of enclosures or a more detailed description. This may be helpful in correspondence from a medical practice when important documents are enclosed. Be sure that the number of enclosures indicated matches the number of items enclosed. Otherwise, readers will be frustrated (or confused) if they feel they did not receive something that should have been enclosed.

The word "Attachment" (also Att:) serves the same purpose as "Enclosure" but usually means that documents are attached by staple or clip.

If additional material is being sent separately, use the term "Separate cover" or "Under separate cover" and identify the item being sent. This notation is also placed at the left margin. An example is as follows:

Under separate cover: *Guide to Treatment of Juvenile Diabetes*

Delivery Identification

Business letters are not always sent by traditional means. When being sent by carriers other than first-class US mail, you may indicate the specific means of delivery after the Enclosure reference or the reference initials, whichever appears last. For example:

By fax
By priority mail
By messenger
By certified mail
By special delivery
By express mail
By e-mail

Avoid the use of the term *via,* which has the potential of being misunderstood by some patients.

Copy Notation

Copy notations let readers know who else will receive the material, which is an important factor in the case of disclosure of protected patient information (PPI). The copy notation serves as a historical record of who has been part of a communication chain and is aware of previous issues, requests, or problems. The symbols vary, sometimes noted as "cc," meaning "carbon copy," or simply "copies" in the plural. Acceptable options are to use:

C: (or c)
CC: (or cc:)
Copy to: (or Copies to)
Distribution:

Use of the colon is optional.

Align the copy identification on the left margin on the second line below the reference initials, enclosure notation, or delivery identification, whichever comes last. Depending on the situation, list the recipients in ranked order or simply in alphabetical order. Titles such as "Mr." or "Mrs." are unnecessary if first names or initials are used with the last names.

Another optional notation is the use of "blind copy" or "bc," indicating that copies are being sent to additional recipients without the addressee's knowledge. Place the "bc" reference on the "blind" copies, but not on the original or the cc's. This might be more appropriate for business letters than correspondence addressed to the patient, since undisclosed distribution is inappropriate for letters containing PPI.

The file copy of the letter should list all blind copy notations (which are usually removed on any other copies made in the future). The writer does not have to personally sign additional copies of the letter. Handwritten notes are sometimes added, however, for explanation.

The assumption is that enclosures are sent with the original letter only, but if enclosures were sent with copies, this should be indicated next to the name of the receiver.

Postscript

Postscripts (ie, PS) are used for afterthoughts or personal comments, and occasionally they are used to add emphasis. You are more likely to see a postscript used in a marketing or personal letter than in a business letter. If used, begin on the third line below the last typed reference or notation, also on the left margin.

CONCLUSION

This chapter takes the approach that preparing business correspondence is not necessarily an area where the administrator and other workers in a medical practice have achieved their highest levels of accomplishment. Even if that premise is false, those charged with communication responsibilities are likely to find something useful for constructing professional letters. If that premise is true, you will find the information in this chapter a helpful reminder and guide for preparing professional letters.

Why should you pay so much attention to the extraneous details outlined in this chapter when primarily you are composing your correspondence to patients about their health care? The answer is simple, whether you are writing your patients to inform, a third-party payer for reimbursement, a bank to obtain a loan, or to register a complaint to a vendor. A well-written letter gains the height of attention from your reader, and your level of professionalism goes a long way in accomplishing your goals as presented. The opposite is also true. Lack of attention to detail is a poor reflection on your practice and will hardly gain the respect and attention that you intend.

chapter 4

The Format of a Professional Communication

As a health care professional, you cannot afford to ignore even the smallest detail of professionalism. And one of the most important avenues for expressing your professionalism is your image. Health care providers generally prefer to reflect a serious persona, which is conveyed by your office décor, layout, order, and cleanliness. The way you present yourself speaks worlds about you. Your professional image is also conveyed by your logo and the way it is used on stationery, letterhead, pamphlets, and brochures. In general, if you want to convey the image of a "no-nonsense" operation, keep your printed materials subdued and businesslike. This doesn't mean boring, however. Use quality paper stock, make your logo prominent, and use boldface type.

Establishing your image is an ongoing process. Any time you distribute printed materials, appear and speak in public, or correspond with a patient, vendor, payer, or lender, you are helping to project and maintain the image you desire. For a physician in practice, or for any health care provider, for that matter, the image you portray helps to establish your authority and to bring credit and respect for the content of the information you are striving to communicate.

The purpose of this chapter is to help you develop and follow patterns that will support your professionalism through neat, clear, concise, accurate, and consistent communiqués. This pertains to letters, memoranda, patient bills, forms, and all other documents that are generated by your medical practice. As an added benefit, once the formats and styles are established, correspondence can be done quickly and knowledge of "the way we do things" can be transferred easily.

FORMATS

Although there are several acknowledged formats that are considered to be professional, you will likely choose what fits your personal style and the layout of your letterhead on your professional stationery.

A business letter must have the appropriate margins, spacing, print font, paragraph length, individual sentence length, and "white space." Balance is important, especially in placement of the text on the page. One frequent error in placement is when short letters are placed too high on the page. The ideal is to place the body of the letter in the center of the page. Longer letters should extend to additional pages, rather than cramming too much into a tight place.

Margins, spacing, and alignment are all factors that create the "first impression" for your letters (and other materials). The objective is to center the letter horizontally on the page with uniform margins.

Top Margins

With letterhead, type the date on the fourth line below the letterhead. On plain paper, type the date on the first line below the 2-inch top margin. Use a one-inch top margin on every continuing page. Letterhead is used only for the first page; pages that follow are either "second sheet" or plain paper.

Bottom Margins

At a minimum, use a bottom margin of one inch. If multiple pages are necessary, increase the bottom margin on the first page to two inches. If your letterhead has printed copy across the bottom, always leave at least a half-inch margin between that and the bottom line of typed copy.

Left and Right Margins

Most computer software has default margins set at 1 inch, although some use 1.25 inches. You may adjust your margin up to 1.75 inches to create a crisp appearance that is easy to read. How much copy your margins and letterhead will accommodate depends on the size of your type font.

Vertical Alignment

A letter of fewer than 100 words typically has eight to ten lines between the date and the inside address. A 100- to 200-word letter typically has six to nine lines between the date and the inside address. Extremely short letters of approximately 50 words call for wide left and right margins.

Multiple-Page Letters

Use plain paper of similar quality (or "second sheets") with identical left and right margins. Type the continuation page heading on the first line below the one-inch margin at the top of the page. Type the name of the recipient, page number, and date, either on one line or on three separate lines. Begin text two lines below the continuation heading. Never carry over the complimentary closing of a business letter to a continuation page. Either adjust the spacing on the first page to allow for the complete text to appear on a single page, or have at least two lines of the body of the letter carry over to the second page. All margins should match the first page. If a page separation splits a paragraph, leave at least two typed lines of the paragraph on the previous page and carry over at least two lines onto the end. Never hyphenate the last word on a page. (See Figure 4-1 for a model of these guidelines.)

STYLES

You may choose from one of the following acceptable formats for setting the style of your correspondence, patient education material, and other documents. Once you have established your own style, use it throughout all your work rather than taking the chance of being inconsistent. It will save preparation time, also, when your defaults are set up in formats that eliminate the decision making.

Extreme (Full) Block Format

The most popular of styles used in word processing is the extreme block format. In this format, all lines begin at the left margin. Only quotations, graphs, tables, and the like are indented. (See Figure 4-1.)

Modified Block (Standard) Format

This format style is identical to the extreme block style except the date, complimentary closing, and signature and title lines are indented to the center of the page. This style, which is business-like, yet friendly, is a popular format.

Modified Block (Indented) Format

With the addition of indentation of one-half inch, or approximately five spaces or one tab space, this style is similar to the modified block (standard) format. It requires more setup time and is the most apt to have formatting errors and inconsistencies.

Simplified Format

In the simplified format, all lines begin at the left margin. The salutation is replaced by a subject line typed in capital letters. The complimentary closing is omitted, and the writer's identification is typed in capital letters on one line following the signature. This format would be very appropriate in writing to companies or organization where the content is about a general policy. One example would be a standard letter to pharmaceutical companies regarding your position on seeing representatives. (See Figure 4-2 for an example of the format as well as sample content.)

READABILITY

A good format contributes to the readability of the letter and communicates a great deal about your professionalism, character, and integrity. Whatever your subject matter and your format, the primary goal of your

FIGURE 4-1

Extreme Block Letter

Intensive Care Clinic of Anytown

127 Healthy Way ■ Anytown, NE ■ 12345
Phone (555) 555-1212
Fax (555) 555-1222

July 31, 2004

REFERENCE: Claim Number 54321

Ms. Wanda Wright
Director, Claims Department
Third-Party Payer Company
66110 East 99th Street
Anytown, NE 12345

Dear Ms. Wright:

SUBJECT: Lack of Timely Payments

For the third month in a row, we have made requests for payment to your claims department personnel. We have not received payment to date, nor have we received a response to previous inquiries. Following up on claims payments is a burden to our busy practice and an aggravation to our staff.

The current amount that Third-Party Payer Company owes Intensive Care Clinic of Anytown for claims that we have filed properly and in a timely manner is $_____.

In the future, unless we receive full payment for services rendered to your policyholders within 30 days of our claims submission to you, we will have no choice but to inform our patients that we will no longer be able to honor their coverage with the Third-Party Payer Company. Since Third-Party Payer Company accounts for 25% of our annual income, we will also have no choice but to suggest alternative coverage to them.

I would appreciate having your response to this letter by August 10, 2004.

Sincerely,

Herbert W. Best, MD
Medical Director

HWB/GMC
By Federal Express
cc: M. R. Wise, MD

Simplified Letter

ABC Medical Center

547 Medical Blvd, Ste 170 • Townsend, TX 77377
Phone (581) 541-1212
Fax (581) 541-1222

Date

Serving Pharmaceutical Company
Vvvvvvvvvvvvv
Vvvvvvvvvvvvvv
Vvvvvvvvvv

POLICY ON VISITS BY PHARMACEUTICAL REPRESENTATIVES

Effective January 1, 2005, ABC Medical Center will see pharmaceutical representatives by appointment only on Tuesdays, Wednesdays, and Thursdays during the hours of 12:00 pm to 1:30 pm.

Please schedule an appointment with the physicians for each of your visits. Appointments will be approximately 10 minutes each.

We hope this system will be more convenient and will decrease your waiting time in the office.

JAMES JONES, PRACTICE ADMINISTRATOR

JJ

correspondence, memorandum, policy, or patient education document is to be readable. That is, your writing must be understandable.

Further, it must be motivating. You want your letter not only to be read, but also to be responded to and acted upon. When you place your written communiqué in the hands of your readers, you are asking them to give it their attention.

To accomplish its purpose, your message must be understood, command attention, persuade the reader, and stay in the reader's mind. These elements may be captured in four key words:

Clarity
Impact
Persuasiveness
Penetration

To accomplish this, consider the following guidelines associated with each of the four words:

- **Clarity.** Use everyday terms to explain medical terminology. Consider your audience when you compose written communication. Say things in the shortest way.

- **Impact.** Peel language back to the bare bones of message. Why is it so difficult to do? It's the way we teach children to talk and write. "This is a dog. See the dog run." Impact language is easy language: easy to write, easy to read, easy to speak, easy to listen to. For maximum impact, tighten sentences around what the subject is or does.

- **Persuasiveness.** All writing is in some sense a sales message. As the transmitter, you want to achieve something, or you wouldn't be going to the trouble of writing or speaking. For the effort to succeed, some degree of agreement, cooperation, or at east response is required on the part of the receivers. To all readerships our job is, simply and clearly, to state facts and—when indicated—say what they mean. When the facts are disagreeable or the news unpleasant, try for "comfortable words." Describe problems, setbacks, new needs, matter-of-factly and even cheerfully. "This is the crisis. This is the danger. This is what has to be done about it. Let's do it!"

- **Penetration.** Concentrate your heaviest firepower on the openings and closings. The opener hooks the reader; the closer sinks the hook. Seek plain and homely figures of speech to reinforce your thought. Make them as picturesque and vivid as you can without losing the parallel. Use picture words. Language can be salted with words having fairly common, fairly predictable, visual connotations.

CONCLUSION

Communications from a physician's practice must represent the professionalism of the practitioner. The most obvious way to accomplish that is through a crisp, neat, and professionally acceptable appearance. Based on the assumption that the technical knowledge of the administrative staff may be somewhat sketchy in terms of "secretarial" skills and more focused on business operations than business letters, this chapter takes a rather basic approach.

Further, since having a sharp look means nothing without substance that the reader can understand, some basic guidelines are also offered for writing with readability in mind.

The next chapters focus on specific examples of letters that work well for or can be adapted to a typical medical practice.

chapter 5

Envelopes, Labels, and Delivery

The problem of delivery of mail and packages is a serious one for medical practices because of the nature of the communication. The incidence of reported nondeliveries seems to be on the rise. One reason that letters and other matter sent by mail fail to arrive is faulty information or incomplete information that patients provide. People move often, and if the demographic information is not obtained *and updated* with every patient visit, the delivery of mail is likely to not succeed.

Aside from the problem of poor information, you can greatly increase the chances of delivery by following certain guidelines established by the United States Postal Service (USPS). Other couriers and delivery services have specific requirements as well. These specifications and other information are the topic of this chapter.

UNITED STATES POSTAL SERVICE

The USPS will be by far your most often-used service provider for corresponding with your patients and vendors. The USPS Web site (http://www.usps.com) is a valuable resource for gaining information and tips on how to best use the mail system. Following are important things to know about how your mail will be viewed and handled, as well as the various services that the USPS offers to its customers.

The USPS guidelines for preparing the delivery address and return address for professional envelopes are outlined in the information that follows.

Delivery Address

The delivery address is the most important information on your mail piece. It specifies where the USPS is to deliver a mail piece. The address must be legible and complete on the side of the mail piece that bears the postage. The address must include:

- Intended recipient's name or other designation
- Delivery address, including street number and name (predirectional, suffix, and postdirectional as appropriate), post office box number, rural or highway contract route and box number, and secondary

descriptor and number (eg, suite or apartment number, floor) if needed

■ City and state

■ ZIP code or ZIP+4 code where required

Use the following format for your delivery addresses:

Name or attention line ⟶ JANE L MILLER
Company ⟶ MILLER ASSOCIATES
Suite or apartment number ⟶ [STE 2006]*
Delivery address ⟶ 1960 WEST CHELSEA AVENUE STE 2006
City, state, ZIP code ⟶ ALLENTOWN PA 18104

Automated mail processing machines read addresses on mail pieces from the bottom up and will first look for a city, state, and ZIP code. Then the machines look for a delivery address. If the machines can't find either line, then your mail piece could be delayed or misrouted. Any information below the delivery address line (a logo, a slogan, or an attention line) could confuse the machines and misdirect your mail.

Prepare your envelopes for mailing using the following guidelines:

■ Always put the address and the postage on the same side of your mail piece.

■ On a letter, the address should be parallel to the longest side.

■ Use all capital letters.

■ Use no punctuation.

■ Use at least ten-point type.

■ Place one space between city and state.

■ Place two spaces between state and ZIP code.

■ Use simple type fonts.

■ Type the address left justified.

■ Use black ink on white or light paper.

■ Don't use reverse type (white printing on a black background).

If your address appears inside a window, make sure there is at least one-eighth-inch clearance around the address. Sometimes parts of the address slip out of view behind the window and mail processing machines can't read the address.

If you are using address labels, make sure you don't cut off any important information. Also make sure your labels are on straight. Mail processing machines have trouble reading crooked or slanted information. (See Figure 5-1 for an example of formatting an envelope.)

---

* If you do not have enough space to include the suite or apartment number on the same line as the delivery address, put it on the line *above* the delivery address, *not* on the line below.

FIGURE 5-1

Addressing an Envelope

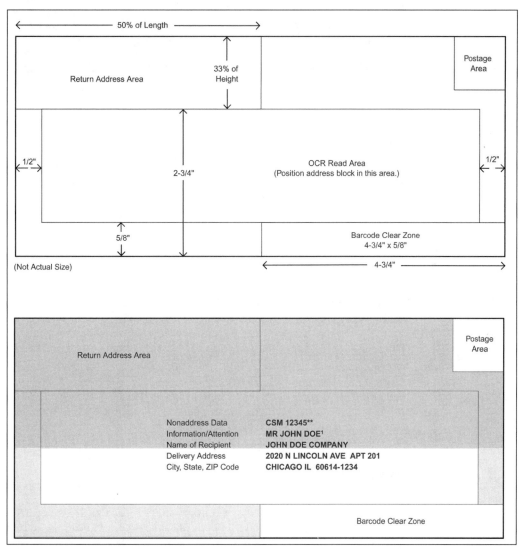

Notes: The name of the recipient must appear in the OCR read area. The darker shaded area indicates "free space" for nonaddress printing. The lighter shaded area indicates preferred clear zone to enhance readability.

The following are some additional tips to remember when addressing pieces intended for mailing:

- Always put the attention line on top, never below the city and state or in the bottom corner of your mail piece.

- If you can't fit the suite or apartment number on the same line as the delivery address, put it on the line *above* the delivery address, *not* on the line below.

- Words like *east* and *west* are called directionals and they are extremely important. A missing or a bad directional can prevent your mail from being delivered correctly.

- Use the free ZIP code lookup and the ZIP+4 code lookup on the USPS Web site to find the correct ZIP codes and ZIP+4 codes for your addresses.

- Almost 25% of all mail pieces have something wrong with the address (eg, a missing apartment number or a wrong ZIP code). Can some of those mail pieces get delivered, in spite of the incorrect address? Yes, but it costs the USPS time and money to do that and your mail will arrive late.

- When a first-class mail letter weighs one ounce or less and the address is parallel to the shortest side, the piece may be nonmailable or will be charged the nonmachineable surcharge.

- Sometimes it's not important that your mail piece reach a specific customer, just that it reach an address. One way to do this is to use a generic title such as "Postal Customer," "Occupant," or "Resident," rather than a name, plus the complete address.

- Fancy type fonts such as those used on wedding invitations do not read well on mail processing equipment. Fancy fonts look great on your envelopes, but also may slow down your mail.

- Use common sense. If you can't read the address, then automated mail processing equipment can't read the address.

- Some types of paper interfere with the machines that read addresses. The paper on the address side should be white or light in color minus patterns or prominent flecks. Also, the envelope shouldn't be too glossy. Avoid shiny, coated paper stock.

Return Address

A return address tells the USPS where the sender wants the mail returned if it is undeliverable. Lots of mailers use a return address because it's an opportunity to "brand" their mail piece with a company name or a logo. The USPS encourages mailers to use return addresses because if the piece is undeliverable they can return it.

The return address has the same elements as the delivery address and must be placed in the upper left corner of the address side or in the upper left of the addressing area.

A return address is required on certain types of mail. Mail qualifying for nonprofit standard mail rates must have the name and return address of the authorized nonprofit organization either on the outside of the mail piece or in a prominent location on the material being mailed (inside the mail piece). Some other instances when mailers *must* use a return address include:

- Paying postage with precanceled stamps
- Priority mail

- Package services
- Mail with special services
- Company permit imprint

Simplified Addressing

Three other types of addressing may apply to mailings from a medical practice. Besides billing statements and professional letters, a practice may also generate mailings as a result of a marketing initiative. The following list provides descriptions of three addressing formats, and Table 5-1 gives additional addressing guidelines.

Simplified addressing: Simplified address format ("Postal Customer") is used when general distribution is requested to each customer on a rural route or highway contract route or to each boxholder at a post office without city carrier service. Government agencies may also use simplified addressing for official matter being sent to all stops on city carrier routes and post office boxholders at post offices with city carrier service.

Occupant addressing: Mailer may use "Occupant" (instead of a recipient's name) with a complete delivery address on mail intended for selective distribution.

Exceptional addressing: Indicates that mail piece should be delivered to the current resident if addressee has moved. Exceptional addressing may not be used on certain types of mail.

Special Address Services (Ancillary Service Endorsements)

Sometimes, no matter how good your address is, USPS still can't deliver the mail. For instance, your patient or addressee may have moved or the

TABLE 5-1

Addressing Guidelines

- Use simple sans serif type with uniform stroke thickness.
- Type or machine-print in dark ink on a light background with a uniform left margin.
- Left-justify every line in the address block.
- Use two-letter state abbreviations.
- Use one space between city and state, two spaces between state and ZIP+4 code.
- Use appropriate ZIP+4 code (if unknown, use five-digit ZIP code).
- You may put logos and slogans on your mail piece, but be careful where you put them. Don't put anything below the delivery line of the delivery address.
- Use eight-point or larger font size for the return address.

Source: USPS Publication 28, *Postal Addressing Standards*

building may be vacant. By using special addressing services, called "ancillary service endorsements," you can give the Postal Service specific instructions for how to handle your mail if it is undeliverable as addressed. Depending on the purpose of your mailing, you may want those pieces forwarded to patients or other addressees who have moved, or you may want a corrected address returned to you. Ancillary service endorsements include four basic phrases that are printed on the address side of your mail piece:

Address Service Requested
Return Service Requested
Change Service Requested
Forwarding Service Requested

Undeliverable mail is handled differently depending on the class of mail, the endorsement you use, and how recently your customer has moved. Some of these actions have fees associated with them and may cost you money.

First-class mail is forwarded free of charge and, if undeliverable, returned to you for free. You can use an ancillary service endorsement to change how your first-class mail is treated. Undeliverable standard mail that doesn't have an endorsement is thrown away by the USPS. This is a good reason to make sure that your address list is correct and current.

And remember these three additional tips:

- Before you put an endorsement on your mail piece, make sure you understand what service you will receive and what fees may be charged for that service.
- Pay special attention to the "weighted fee" charge for standard mail endorsed "Address Service Requested" or "Forwarding Service Requested." This fee more than doubles the original postage cost and catches many mailers by surprise.
- The best way to avoid undeliverable or returned pieces is to check the accuracy of your address list *before* you mail.

Permits and Postage

You may want to do mailings to introduce a new service or for various marketing purposes. The USPS has three different ways for you to pay postage for bulk mailings. This section will help you choose the payment method that's right for you.

There are three steps:

1. Choose a method of postage payment.
   a. Precanceled stamps
   b. Postage meters
   c. Permit imprints
2. Get a mailing permit.
3. Pay an annual mailing fee.

Precanceled Stamps

Precanceled stamps allow you to apply stamps to your mail pieces. With precanceled stamps, you affix a lower rate of postage and then pay the difference when you drop off your mailing. Stamps add a personal touch to your envelope and may give your addressee an added incentive to open and read your mail.

Postage Meter

A postage meter prints postage directly onto your mail pieces or onto a meter tape, which you apply to your mail piece (see Figure 5-2). Postage meters are a very convenient way to pay for postage and track postage costs for your practice or organization.

Some mailers use metered postage because they believe that it adds a more personal touch. A postage meter is also great to have around the office for all of your mailing needs. You can send out any class of mail (except periodicals) in any quantity at any rate with the same postage meter.

Postage meters come in all sizes. Very large mailers have big, specialized meters that fold, stuff, weigh, and meter postage onto envelopes. Some meters are small and require each mail piece to be hand-fed. A meter manufacturer can help you decide which meter is right for your mailing needs.

If you already have a postage meter and you're starting to do bulk mailing, using your meter is a smart choice. Although you can use the same postage meter for all of your mail, you must apply for a permit to use the meter for bulk mailings. Also, there are special markings required for bulk mailings that can be applied with your meter stamp. That saves you an extra step.

Permit Imprint

Permit imprint is the most popular and convenient way to pay for postage, especially for high-volume mailings. Instead of using precanceled stamps or a postage meter, the mailer prints postage information in the upper right corner of the mail piece. This postage block is called an *indicia* (see Figure 5-3). The indicia is printed onto each mail piece.

To use permit imprint, you set up a postage account (called an "advance deposit account") at the post office where you'll be depositing your mail. When you bring your mailing to the post office, the total

F IGURE 5 - 2

Postage From a Postage Meter

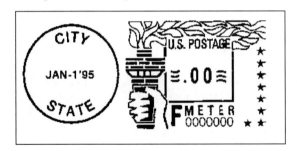

FIGURE 5-3

Permit Imprint Indicia

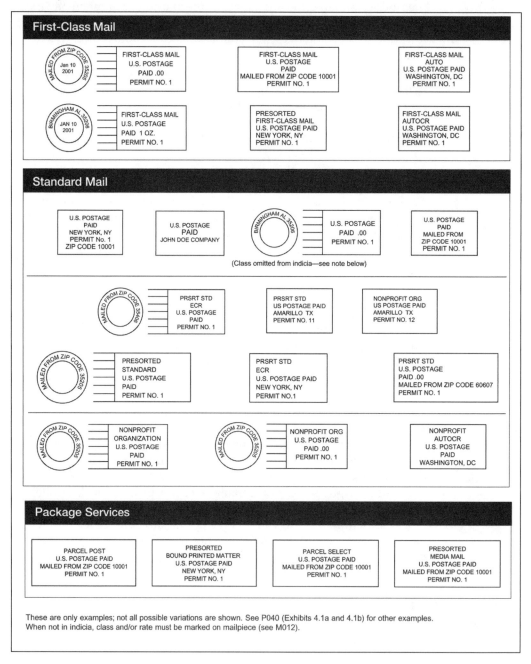

These are only examples; not all possible variations are shown. See P040 (Exhibits 4.1a and 4.1b) for other examples.
When not in indicia, class and/or rate must be marked on mailpiece (see M012).

postage is deducted from your account. It's like having a checking account at the post office.

The key to permit imprint is identical-weight pieces. All of your mail pieces must weigh exactly the same. Permit imprint is simple and convenient; you save time because you're not affixing postage to each piece. You print the permit imprint when you print the rest of your mail piece.

If you already have a mail piece printed without the permit imprint, you can use a rubber stamp.

Permit imprint is convenient because you don't have to buy postage in advance, remember to reset your meter, or worry about putting the right amount of postage on each piece.

Additional Resources for Business Mailers

The USPS has many different people and tools that can help you with all aspects of your mailing. All of these services are available free of charge.

- There is a 24-hour information hotline: **1-800-ASK-USPS**
- Customer service representatives can answer all of your questions about the USPS and your mail:
  http://www.usps.com/ncsc/locators/find-pbc.html
- Postmasters are in daily contact with customers and can advise you who to call with questions about your mail:
  http://www.usps.com/ncsc/locators/find-po.html

USPS Terminology

When dealing with the USPS, you may encounter words and phrases that seem familiar but are not readily understood. The following is a list of those terms and their definitions as they apply to the USPS.

Advance deposit account: A debit account into which a mailer deposits funds that are maintained by the USPS and from which postage is deducted at the time of mailing.

Automation-compatible mail: Mail that can be scanned and processed by automated mail processing equipment such as a bar code sorter.

Balloon rate: A rate charged for priority mail and parcel post items that weigh less than 15 pounds and measure more than 84 inches but no more than 108 inches in combined length and girth.

Bulk mail: The term generally used to describe presorted first-class mail and standard mail.

Bulk mail center (BMC): A highly mechanized mail processing plant that distributes standard mail in piece and bulk form.

Business mail entry unit (BMEU): The area of a postal facility where mailers present bulk, presorted, and permit mail for acceptance. The BMEU includes dedicated platform space, office space, and a staging area on the workroom floor.

Carrier route presort mail: Mail sorted by carrier route to qualify for discount postage rates. The mail requires no primary or secondary distribution. The term is a general descriptor of the available rates for this type of preparation, which includes enhanced carrier route standard mail, automation carrier route first-class mail, carrier route periodicals, and carrier route bound printed matter.

Destination entry discount: A postage discount for depositing mail at specific postal facilities (eg, delivery unit or bulk mail center) that are closer to the final destination of the mail.

Full letter tray: A tray filled at least three-fourths full with faced, upright pieces. Each tray must be physically filled to capacity before the filling of the next tray. A tray with less mail may be prepared only if less-than-full or overflow trays are permitted by the standards for the rate claimed.

Indicia: Imprinted designation on mail that denotes postage payment (eg, permit imprint).

Known office of publication: The business office of a periodicals publication that is in the city where the original entry for periodicals mailing privileges is authorized.

Mailing permit: Permission to mail at bulk (presorted) rates.

Meter tape: A piece of adhesive paper that is fed through a postage meter and imprinted with postage. The meter tape is then applied to a mail piece (usually a large envelope or parcel that is too big to fit through the postage meter).

Nonmachinable surcharge: A surcharge applied to mail pieces that cannot be sorted on mail processing equipment because of size, shape, content, or address legibility. Such mail must be processed manually.

Oversized rate: Parcel post rate for pieces exceeding 108 inches but not more than 130 inches in combined length and girth.

Permit imprint: Printed indicia, instead of an adhesive postage stamp or meter stamp, that shows postage prepayment by an authorized mailer.

Postage meter: A device that can print one or more denominations of postage onto a mail piece or meter tape. It is available for lease only from designated manufacturers.

Presort: The process by which a mailer prepares mail so that it is sorted to the finest extent required by the standards for the rate claimed. Generally, presort is performed sequentially, from the lowest (finest) level to the highest level, to those destinations specified by standard and is completed at each level before the next level is prepared. Not all presort levels are applicable to all mailings.

Presorted first-class mailing: A nonautomation rate category for a mailing that consists of at least 500 addressed mail pieces and is sorted and prepared according to USPS standards. This mail does not bear a bar code.

Presorted mail: A form of mail preparation, required to bypass certain postal operations, in which the mailer groups pieces in a mailing by ZIP code or by carrier route or carrier walk sequence (or other USPS–recommended separation).

Presorted rates: A discounted postage rate. In exchange for this lower postage rate, mailers must sort their mail into containers based on the ZIP code destinations on the mail.

Residual shape surcharge: A surcharge applied to standard mail pieces that are prepared as parcels or that are not letter size or flat size (eg, mailing tubes).

Sectional center facility (SCF): A postal facility that serves as the processing and distribution center (P&DC) for post offices in a designated geographic area as defined by the first three digits of the ZIP codes of those offices. Some SCFs serve more than one three-digit ZIP code range.

Single-piece rate: The "undiscounted" or "full" postage rate available for individual pieces of Express Mail, First–Class Mail, Priority Mail, and Package Services. Single-piece rates contrast with rates available for presorted mail.

Sort: To separate mail by a scheme or ZIP code range; to separate and place mail into a carrier case; to distribute mail by piece, package, bundle, sack, or pouch.

Sortation: The distribution or separation of mail to route it to its final delivery point.

Weighted fee: The fee charged the sender for standard mail pieces endorsed "Address Service Requested" or "Forwarding Service Requested" that are returned as undeliverable. The fee equals the single-piece first-class mail rate multiplied by a factor of 2.472 and then rounded to the next whole cent.

Zoned rate: A rate structure for certain priority mail, periodicals (except nonadvertising portion), and package services (parcel post and bound printed matter) that is based on weight and distance traveled (or zones crossed).

USPS Calendar

In addition to closing on Sundays, the USPS observes the following holidays and, therefore, does not operate on these days:

Martin Luther King, Jr's Birthday
Washington's Birthday (Presidents' Day)
Memorial Day
Independence Day
Labor Day
Columbus Day
Veterans Day
Thanksgiving Day
Christmas Day
New Year's Day

Special Delivery Options

For times you want to send your mail with added convenience or greater security, USPS offers a variety of services to meet your needs. Whether it's a receipt, a verification of delivery, or payment upon delivery, USPS' extra services—Delivery Confirmation, Signature Confirmation, etc—add flexibility to all of the ways you mail or ship.

Delivery Confirmation service gives you the date, ZIP code, and time that your article was delivered. If delivery was attempted, you will get the date and time of attempted delivery. You can easily access this information online. Although several options for delivery confirmation are available through USPS, those particularly applicable to the medical practice include:

- **First-class mail parcels:** Envelopes and small packages weighing 13 ounces or less. Applies only to boxes or envelopes measuring at least three fourths of an inch at the thickest point.
- **Priority Mail®:** Cost-effective delivery in an average of two to three days.
- **Package services parcels:** Small and large packages, envelopes, and tubes. Includes Parcel Post®, media mail, bound printed matter, and library mail.

You can use Delivery Confirmation with the following extra services:

- **Return receipt for merchandise:** Provides a mailing receipt and a return receipt with the date of delivery and the recipient's signature.
- **Insured mail:** Insurance against loss or damage for merchandise and gifts.
- **Registered mail:** Provides maximum security and date of delivery or attempted delivery.
- **Return receipt:** Provides a postcard with the date of delivery and recipient's signature.
- **Restricted delivery:** Confirms that only a specified person (or authorized agent) will receive a piece of mail. Only available with certified mail, insured mail greater than $50, or Registered Mail.

The USPS also offers customers the ability to print shipping labels via the Internet and the option to purchase shipping supplies (eg, boxes, envelopes, forms) online.

OTHER CARRIERS

Other carriers (eg, DHL, Federal Express, and United Parcel Service) provide services similar to the USPS that offer delivery options to the medical practice. In addition to couriers and delivery services that you may use in your local area, you may find the services of the following other companies appropriate for various types of deliveries for your business operations. Standard features such as tracking and next day and second day delivery are features that appeal to the needs of the business office. Information is available online at the following addresses:

DHL: http://www.dhl-usa.com/home/home.asp
Federal Express: http://www.fedex.com/us/
United Parcel Service: http://www.ups.com

National and international couriers and delivery services, such as those listed, are very competitive in their pricing and in the services they offer. Obtain bids and price lists periodically from each vendor to compare current rates and options that best meet the needs of your practice.

CONCLUSION

Getting your correspondence delivered is the objective of this chapter. Not only is it important to have the correct address information and to place it in the specified location on the envelope, you must also send it in the best way to achieve your goal. The USPS and other delivery carriers offer many services to make your job easier. The information in this chapter is provided to you as a resource for your various mailing needs.

Common Letters

Letters and memos with various tones and objectives are used for many occasions in the medical practice. This chapter explores typical letters appropriate for sending and examples of how these would be constructed by using the principles of writing techniques and formatting that are covered in the previous chapters. Some of the same content and guidelines for development would also apply to memorandums. More about writing effective memorandums will be discussed in Chapter 7.

INTRODUCTIONS

Letters of introduction are used on many occasions in the medical practice. They should always be written in a positive and persuasive tone to stimulate the reader to finish reading the correspondence. One application of an introduction letter would be to introduce a new associate. This type of communiqué need not be lengthy, but it should include the name, position, and date of employment (or effective date of the association). It should provide the background information that validates the associate's education, experience, and previous position. Finally, it should also stress the importance of the relationship.

Figure 6-1 is an example of an introduction letter that could be used to introduce a new associate to your patients, your colleagues, the medical community, your staff, and others.

Another example of an introduction letter is to introduce a change in procedures. Applications to the medical practice would be to notify your patients of changes in billing processes, telephone service, office hours, etc. Again, using a positive and persuasive tone, you would draft a letter to introduce the change, explain the previous process, describe the change and convey benefits, and offer assistance. The letter in Figure 6-2 introduces a change in your practice procedures.

Other examples of letters introducing change are to announce new office locations or to present a new product or service (see the upcoming section regarding marketing letters). A new location introduction should have the following components and details:

■ Announcement of location
  —Address
  —Phone numbers

Figure 6-1

Introduction Letter for a New Associate

PRN Medical Associates

1311 River Exchange Drive
Atlanta, GA 30077
707 543-2218
707 543-2228 (fax)

[date]

[inside address]

Dear Dr. [name]:

On behalf of PRN Medical Associates, I am happy to announce that, effective September 1, 2004, Dr. Major Brown will be joining our staff in the specialty of [name of specialty]. Dr. Brown will begin seeing patients on that date.

A graduate of [college or university] with a [degree] in [subject], Dr. Brown received his doctorate from [medical school], where he graduated with honors. He completed his residency program in [name of specialty] at [name of institution]. Most recently, he has practiced in [name of city] since completing his training.

Our practice will be greatly enhanced with the addition of Dr. Brown. Dr. Brown will be calling you in the next few weeks to introduce himself and to schedule a time to meet with you. I know you will like Major and will help make him feel welcome as soon as you meet him. Thank you in advance for this kindness.

Sincerely,

[name], MD

KS

FIGURE 6-2

Introduction Letter for a New Telephone System

PRN Medical Associates

1311 River Exchange Drive
Atlanta, GA 30077
707 543-2218
707 543-2228 (fax)

[date]

Dear Patients:

In our commitment to improve our service to you, we have changed our telephone system to better respond to your needs.

Previously, your telephone calls have been answered by a live attendant and your call directed to the appropriate person to answer your needs. Because of the heavier flow of incoming calls at some times over others, it has been difficult for all your calls to be handled promptly and for your call to be transferred quickly.

To handle more calls, we have installed an automated attendant telephone service. This system will enable you to get to your intended party without being put on hold or waiting for your call to be answered, which sometimes occurs when the call traffic exceeds what our staff can handle. We believe with the automated attendant you will experience quicker and smoother access by directing your call yourself through the selections available. Or, if you prefer, you may always select "0" to get an operator.

Our telephone number remains the same. If you have any questions about telephone access to the practice, please call us at 707 543-2218. We appreciate your selecting our practice for your health care, and we look forward to serving you in the future.

Sincerely,

[name], MD

KS

       —Driving directions
- Benefits to reader
  - —Closer proximity to patient base
  - —Proximity to other providers
  - —Larger facility
- Explanation of service
  - —Days, hours, etc
  - —Types of patient services provided
- More benefits
  - —Additional parking available
  - —Proximity to public transportation
- Close with invitation

These are merely a few of the types of letters and examples of information you will use in your practice to make an announcement of something new. Remember the guidelines to be positive in tone, succinct in your sentence structure, and professional in your formatting.

THANK YOU

Saying "thank you" in writing is appropriate for many instances in a medical practice and comes easily to most writers. Whether you are thanking a medical director of a hospital, a professional colleague, a patient, an employee, a vendor, or someone who has extended special service or a favor, the most important points are to be specific and to be sincere. Being timely in expressing thanks is also significant. Following are some examples of applications for your practice.

- **Meeting.** Open with appreciation for granting the meeting. (An example would be a meeting with a hospital medical director about a matter of concern or with a professional colleague about a potential partnership.) Refer specifically to the event. Convey appreciation for the time invested. Make a personal comment about a specific statement that was made during the meeting. Close with a pleasant statement.

- **Hospitality.** Open with thanks about the event or kindness. Be sincere and specific about what you appreciated. Close with a pleasant comment.

- **Invitation.** Begin by acknowledging the invitation. Accept or decline with graciousness. If declining, consider offering a brief explanation. End on a positive note.

- **Assistance.** Convey a genuine tone throughout. Begin with a personal comment. Be specific in explaining how the reader assisted you. Close with a thank you or expression of gratitude.

- **Appreciation.** Express gratitude about the incident or thoughtfulness. State your sincere appreciation. End with a pleasant comment.

- **Support.** Open with a thank-you for the expression of support. Be specific about the incident or action to which you are referring. Announce the outcome or expected outcome of the support. Convey appreciation again. Close with a message of goodwill.

- **Patient referral.** Open with a thank you for the referral. Be specific about the patient or subject involved. Announce the outcome or expected outcome of the referral. State your plan of action for follow-up communication. Close with a goodwill message.

- **Gifts.** Be brief and sincere. Open by expression of appreciation. Describe a specific use of or benefit from the gift. End with a pleasant remark.

The principles of being genuine and specific when writing thank-you letters and memos to express appreciation apply equally to those addressed to internal and external readers.

REQUESTS

In your medical practice, you will have many opportunities to write letters of request, such as the following partial list:

- Request for forms, information, explanation, etc
- Request for books, periodicals, information
- Request for patient consultation
- Request for care
- Requests for insurance information and participation status
- Request for office equipment bids
- Requests for computer hardware or software proposals (RFPs)
- Request for service

An ideal letter of request will have the following components:

- Your request (open with a specific explanation of the information you need, the order you are placing, etc)
- All relevant information (ie, amounts, names, dates, etc)
- Your reason for the request
- A deadline for the response
- Contact information to which the reader can direct a response
- A closing that states your appreciation for the reader's help

Figure 6-3 is an example of a letter of request that can be easily adapted to various uses.

FIGURE 6-3

Letter of Request

John Doe, MD

437 Park Place
Madison, WI 79228
909 707 5432
909 707-5442 (fax)

[date]

[inside address]

Dear [Name of Insurance Company]:

In August 2004, I plan to open a medical practice in Madison, Wisconsin. It is my understanding that your company offers various types of insurance coverage for medical practices.

I am particularly interested in receiving information on malpractice insurance coverage. I would also appreciate learning about other appropriate business indemnifications that I may need and welcome the advice of an experienced broker for my general insurance needs.

Please contact me to arrange a time that is convenient to meet to discuss these vital matters, preferably by June 15, 2004. My telephone number is 909 707-5432, and I am also available by cell phone at 909 685-6459.

Thank you for your assistance. I look forward to your call.

Sincerely,

[name], MD

JD

In addition to sending letters of request, you will also have occasion to respond to requests from your peers, patients, business associates, and others. In this case, in the ideal letter you will thank the reader for the request, explain what you can do, and conclude by offering future assistance (if feasible) or expressing appreciation.

When you have to decline a request, open your letter on a positive note, give a reason(s) for the refusal, give the actual refusal, and if possible, offer alternatives. It is important to be tactful and considerate throughout the letter.

ANNOUNCEMENTS

Announcement letters are similar to introduction letters and can follow the same format. You might use an announcement letter to announce a move to a new location. In this instance, you would state your announcement; note the new address and telephone number; describe the benefits of the move; and close with an invitation to call or visit the new location.

From time to time, you may have to announce something that is not so pleasant. In this case, the ideal letter will have a positive tone; announce the change; explain the reasons for the change; emphasize the benefits of your practice and services; and close with a goodwill message.

MARKETING

Some physicians find it difficult to market themselves or their practices through traditional methods used in other business environments. Nevertheless, when you have professional services to offer and products that will benefit your patients, how will they know about them if you do not get the word out? The objective is to introduce yourself and your services in a style that befits the professionalism of your practice.

The well-written marketing letter would have the following components:

- An attention-getting statement

  Do you need more minutes in your day? Now you can receive the same personal health care for your family—but closer to your home—and at more available hours.

- Description of the service or product

  PRN Medical Associates is opening a brand new satellite office in your neighborhood, with expanded office hours. Through our new open-access scheduling, we will see you on the day of your choice.

- Short paragraphs, short sentences, and bulleted lists for visual appeal

  All you need is to call ahead or come in, and you will:
  - Be seen by the physician or nurse practitioner
  - Get prescription refills

■ Benefits (as opposed to features)

Just think of it. No more driving in traffic or adjusting your schedule to make an appointment days or weeks out. Instead, excellent health care is readily available near your home.

■ More benefits

And the best part is that, as an existing patient, your medical records are always available. That's right, no waiting, and no preplanning. Our providers will be ready to see you when you need to be seen.

■ Response information

All you need to do is to come to our satellite office at

800 Willow Road Center
Suite A
Suburbanville, GA
707 589-9900

■ A request for action

All you need to do is call or drop in, and we will take care of you promptly. So when you are not feeling well or you have a health concern, come in to our new office.

The marketing letter that is becoming to a medical practice or health care provider should be attention-getting but not trite, stress benefits, give information, and request action.

APOLOGY

Apologies are in order when misunderstandings occur, expectations are not met, or poor service is delivered. In writing letters of apology, some basic guidelines apply that, when followed, increase your chances of relieving the hard feelings that may result from these circumstances. Following are some points to remember as you put your thoughts in writing:

■ Use a warm and sincere tone

■ Explain the mistake/misunderstanding

■ Acknowledge the inconvenience

■ Apologize

■ Offer specific explanations

■ Avoid making excuses

■ If possible, explain how the issue will be resolved

■ Discuss any follow-up needed at this point

■ Offer your help if needed

■ Close sincerely

Some people find it tempting to apologize while only accepting partial responsibility. This attitude is shown by a critical tone, a condescending air, and reluctant assistance. This type of communication will only incite more hard feelings.

Incidences arise when, indeed, you are only partially responsible for the outcome. However, you should still apologize, but strive for a positive outcome. When writing a letter that accepts partial responsibility, attempt to do the following:

- Be sincere
- Validate the concern, even if you are not fully responsible for the problem
- Offer your unique perspective about the circumstances
- Show your interest and empathy
- Be careful about admitting liability in the event it may affect future actions your reader may take
- Emphasize anything that you can do to alleviate the situation; state action steps that will correct the problem
- Express your goodwill and the importance of the relationship to you

A well-written letter of apology, expressed sincerely, will go a long way to smooth ruffled feathers and minimize conflict in your professional relationships.

EMPLOYMENT

The ideal employment letter will encompass the following:

- Highlight—don't restate exactly—key elements of your resume or curriculum vitae
- Express that you want the job
- State why you are the best candidate for the position
- Ask for an interview
- Describe your action steps

Before you send a letter seeking a position, check it for grammatical errors, typographical mistakes, and misspelled words.

PROPOSALS

Although writing proposals may not be a part of your everyday routine, you may be called upon to submit proposals for various projects or assignments from time to time. More likely, you will receive proposals more often than write them. A well-organized proposal letter will have an introduction, a statement of the issues, a proposed approach to the project, professional fees, resources available (ie, who will be doing the work), agreement and payment terms, mutual indemnifications, and references. Finally, the proposal will have a means for execution of the agreement, usually signature and date lines as validation of acceptance. Depending on the nature of the work, the arrangement should be covered by a privacy policy in compliance with the Health Insurance Portability and Accountability Act of 1996.

REQUEST FOR PROPOSALS

Requests for proposals (RFPs) or requests for quotes (RFQs) are helpful tools for collecting information from vendors. The purpose of an RFP is to ask questions that will get parallel answers so that you can compare "apples to apples" when evaluating products or equipment. The ideal RFP will have the following components:

- Introduction

  Family Health Center is a medical practice with 6 physicians and 15 staff employees. We would like to receive proposals that offer services to include planning, installation, and service for the following project.

- Due date: State the specific time and date that is your deadline to receive a written response

- Project: Describe what you want to accomplish

  Replacement of current Macintosh computer Appletalk network to PC-based Windows NT.

- Current equipment. In this section, describe your current computer system, eg, number of computers, printers, wiring, Internet access, Web site, software, etc, and also the age of your system and any problems you are having.

  Current Computer System

  Number of computers: 25

  System

  Number of printers: 4 (black and white)

  Network wiring: 3-prong telephone wiring

  Internet access: one computer has 28.8 modem

  Web site: for medical students seeking residency information

  Software: all pre-1993 software

  Age of Current System

  Twenty computers are 9 years old; five computers are 4 years old; Printers: 4 to 9 years old, black and white only

  Hardware of Current System

  Present day software will not run or runs too slowly on current computer hardware

- Equipment needs: Define the problem you are trying to solve and what equipment you need to solve it

  New computer system to perform the following functions:

  - Internet access
  - Internet e-mail and interoffice e-mail
  - Voice recognition dictation to reduce dictation expenses

- Track hospital patients (patient lists)
- Presentation software
- Home access to computer system (dial-in access)
- Use of up-to-date continuing medical education programs

Computers:

- *1 server.* Pentium II, 450 MHz, 512 MB RAM, Monitor, 8GB hard drive, 40X CD ROM drive, ethernet 10/100 Base T network card, etc. NT server license
- *20 Desktop Machines.* Pentium II, at least 400 MHz, 96 MB RAM, monitor 4-6GB hard drive, 40X CD ROM drive, Creative Labs Soundblaster 16 sound card, Ethernet 10/100 network card.
- *5 Laptops.* Pentium II, 333 MHz, 128 MB RAM, Ethernet 10/100 Base T network card, Creative Labs Soundblaster 16 sound card, CD-ROM drive, etc
- *Backup devices.* Tape drive backup devices and software
- Other equipment. Scanner and software; 25 Palm Pilot V; 2 Ethernet hubs 10/100 Base T – 16 ports; 6 laser printers
- *Software.* Office and Internet e-mail; Dragon Dictate (Medical Suite); Microsoft Office 2000 software suite; Database Software, probably Filemaker Pro 5.0; antivirus programs; dial-in access
- *Other expenses.* ISP (Internet service provider) monthly fee; wiring for ethernet fees; system equipment installation; yearly maintenance fee for service contract.

■ Installation: Give date for completion.

■ Training: Ask for training information, including pricing, number of people, etc

■ Essential features: Here is where you will ask specific questions depending on what you are trying to accomplish with your purchase.

An RFP is applicable to any kind of equipment; and, although it takes some planning to develop, it will help you immeasurably in getting the information that you need to purchase wisely.

CREDIT ADJUSTMENTS

You will find yourself on both sides of the fence in having to issue credit adjustments and also having to request credit adjustments, from time to time. The ideal letter will bear in mind how you would like to be treated on either side of the problem.

In some cases your patient will notify you of a billing error or other discrepancy, but at other times, your office will discover an error. Validating the discovery in writing is appropriate. Your letter should be specific about what error occurred; present an apology; provide facts about what steps you have taken to remedy the situation; and offer your availability to address problems in the future, if they arise.

If you experience a billing error from a vendor, your letter should identify the specific error; ask for an immediate correction; maintain a neutral rather than a critical tone; provide facts (dates, dollar amounts, account numbers, check/credit card numbers, documentation on previous calls or letters you have exchanged); and, if possible, state a benefit to the vendor/seller of eliminating future errors.

COMPLAINTS

You will have to write letters to complain on various occasions, as well. One example is for misunderstanding of instructions. Another is for lack of courtesy or unsatisfactory performance of an employee, product, or service. An important point for construction of a letter of complaint is to identify the problem, being clear about what is unsatisfactory. Use a pleasant tone, providing appropriate facts without attacking. State your expectations or requirements and ask for an immediate correction. You may also add other action steps that will be beneficial. If you are going to pursue your complaint further, inform the reader of your intended actions (if applicable). End every letter with a word of appreciation.

COLLECTION

Collection letters, the bane of every medical practice, usually occur in "degrees" of intervention. An unpleasant task at any degree, the objective is to get paid for your services while maintaining your professional posture. Remember these guidelines for the various stages of reminders when developing your series of collection letters:

1. **Gentle reminder.** Assume the patient has sent a payment that crossed in the mail; use positive language; remind the patient of the specifics (ie, date, amount, etc); close with a thank you.
2. **Stronger reminder.** Using positive language, remind the patient of the importance of good credit, and ask if there is a problem of which you are unaware. Offer to help, but restate the need to send the payment immediately.
3. **Third reminder.** Using stern but professional language, remind the reader of the overdue amount and send the message that you wish to collect the balance immediately. Avoid any hint of threat, which would be entirely inappropriate. Ask for the reason for the nonpayment. Set a deadline for payment or a call of explanation. For example,

   Please remit your unpaid balance or call us by the close of business on November 30, 2004, to clarify this matter.
4. **Fourth reminder.** Using stern language, restate the reminder of the past due amount. Mention that more serious action will be necessary if the situation is not resolved. Establish a deadline for receipt of the amount. This letter should be kept short.
5. **Final call for payment (with stated consequences).** Briefly review the record of attempts to receive payment, using severe but businesslike language. State the specific consequences of failure to pay by a set deadline. Nevertheless, leave the door open for your patient to return by mentioning that you regret the turn of events.

Although your practice collection policy may differ from this progression, you will still need to adhere to these letter-writing principles in whatever stage your past due balances are in.

SYMPATHY

It is appropriate to send a letter of condolence for the loss of a spouse, parent, or child. Begin with a sincere and comforting expression of sympathy. Give a personal recollection of the person who has died. End with an offer of help and additional condolences.

CONCLUSION

One characteristic holds true throughout every example given in this chapter: the need to be sincere. Other common traits are brevity, clarity, and professionalism. Using these skills and pointers, you will be able to generate effective letters and communications that accomplish your goals and reflect well on your practice.

Effective Memos

Memorandums have a definite place in the medical practice, but they are often written poorly and used incorrectly. Memos are generally intended to be internal communications used to manage the information flow in organizations. The paper memo is slowly being replaced by electronic mail, which is by far the most prevalent way for people within an organization to communicate with each other. The trend toward e-mail will continue.

The tone of memorandums from your medical practice will reflect your practice's culture. Memos can be written in a businesslike tone or a personal tone, depending upon whether you want your message to convey formality or warmth. The subject matter will also govern whether the style or nature is formal or casual.

Memos are useful for announcements, news, meeting notices, policies, requests, responses, and reminders that must be communicated to individuals and groups within your organization. If the content of the memo is confidential, this should be noted above the heading.

You may want to establish a format that is specific to your practice, but if not, you may use the following general guidelines. The important point is to be consistent and professional, even though memorandums are for your internal use. The more professional you are in your approach, the more respect you will gain for the information that you are communicating. The more readable your memo, the more likely you are to get buy-in from your readers.

FORMATS

Your word processing software will automatically set up memo formats for you. Most programs have a pull-down menu that gives you several options for styles, margins, and headings. You can access these formats when you want to open a new document. You can also develop your own format with some link to your practice specialty, mission, or culture. Because it is your internal communication method, you are free to choose.

Figures in this chapter use various styles (ie, professional, contemporary, and elegant) of memos as example formats. (See Figure 7-1 for a sample of the contemporary style and Figure 7-2 for the professional style.)

F I G U R E   7 - 1

Memo Notifying of a Meeting

Memorandum

To: All Staff Members

CC: Drs. Brown, Green, and White

From: Shirley Black, Practice Administrator

Date: 2/7/05

Re: Staff Meeting, Monday, February 14, 2005, 7:30 AM

We will have a staff meeting on Monday, February 14, 2005, at 7:30 a.m., in the break room. Since EMR software is being implemented within the next few weeks, our agenda will focus on changes to work flow processes. To prepare for this meeting, please come with a list of your daily work routines. We will discuss ways other practices have implemented changes and recommendations by our technology consulting firm.

At the conclusion of this meeting, you will be able to anticipate how the implementation of EMR will affect you and what you can anticipate will be your primary challenges during the transition. Since we have a full agenda for this meeting, we won't take time for other matters but will address other issues in the following week's staff meeting.

See you on Monday!

Memo

ABC Medical Practice, PA

To: ABC Staff Members
From: Shirley Black, Practice Administrator
CC: Drs. Brown, Green, and White
Date: June 14, 2004
Re: Changes in Policy on Request for Paid Time Off (PTO)

Effective September 1, 2004, ABC Medical Practice will institute the following policy for request for paid time off (PTO). This is in response to recent confusion about the process for requesting PTO and some overlap in absences that resulted in staffing shortages. The objective is clarification and represents a refinement of the policy that is currently in place. The management team believes that these changes will boost morale and increase productivity.

Requesting PTO with sufficient advance notice allows for consideration of staffing coverage and assessment of operations. Since it is essential for the managers to evaluate staffing based upon anticipated operating requirements during the proposed period of absence, the following guidelines must be followed for the good of all.

- All employees should use PTO during the year it is accrued.
- Requests should be made two weeks in advance of the leave.
- Supervisors should notify each other of staff scheduling and coordinate their schedules to maximize operational efficiencies.
- Employees may not use PTO to supplement a shortage of hours to complete a 40-hour work week.
- PTO must be approved in writing by a supervisor prior to the date of leave. Forms are available in the business office.
- PTO for illnesses must be accounted for as a house-confining illness, a medical evaluation, or other criteria known to and approved by the supervisor.

If you have any questions or concerns about any aspect of the PTO policy, check with your supervisor or me. Your time off is important to you to get rest and relaxation and pursue your outside interests, which are vital for employee satisfaction.

The management staff is convinced that using your PTO wisely and requesting time off in advance will benefit everyone as a whole. Let's commit to following these guidelines so all of us can enjoy the time off we have earned and so that no one is left carrying more than their share of the workload.

Headings

The size of your organization will determine the level of detail that you will use. For example, a large clinic or hospital will use identifiers such as "Department," "Floor No.," "Phone No.," and "Fax No.," while these would be unnecessary in a small to medium-sized practice.

Always type the headings in uppercase letters (even in bold print), with each item followed by a colon. Titles like "Mr.", "Mrs.", and "Ms." are not used in memos. In very casual memos, first names only are appropriate.

Example of headings:

DATE: February 7, 2005
TO: Administrative Staff
FROM: Jane Jones
RE: Staff Meeting, February 14, 2005, 7:30 AM
CC: Drs. Brown, Green, and White

Body of the Memo

Use the following guidelines to format the body of the memo:

- Start typing three lines below the last heading.
- Do not place a salutation in the body of the memo.
- Type memos single-spaced, and align all lines to the left margin, or indent one-half inch on the first line of each paragraph.
- Leave one blank line between paragraphs.
- Memos do not normally require a signature line because they tell who generated the memo in the headings.
- Hand-write the initials of the sender next to the typed name in the heading.
- Optional notations, if used, are to be placed in the following order:
  —Reference initials
  —File notation
  —Enclosure notation
  —Copy notation (if different from the distribution list shown at the top of the memo)
- Confidential notation, if needed, is typed in bold print and uppercase letters three lines below the heading and three lines above the body of the memo.
- If continuing pages are necessary, use the same style as outlined in the formats for letters in Chapter 4.

READABILITY

As in letters and other correspondence, in memos readability is essential to getting your message across. In addition to the principles of good writing expressed in earlier chapters, use these tips for writing memos that are easy to read and understand.

- Use short paragraphs to achieve fast action
- Use subheadings to identify blocks of information to help readers skim the material
- Use white space to improve the appearance of your memo
- Check your spelling for accuracy to increase your credibility
- Answer the questions of "who, what, where, when, why, and how" to cover the bases of what the reader will ask
- Avoid acronyms, jargon, and buzz talk to avoid clouded meanings
- Create a positive tone wherever possible and, likewise, avoid sarcasm. Never use a memo to vent your frustrations
- Be short, simple, and to the point
- Use down-to-earth language, and avoid technical or legalistic verbiage
- As with any written document or correspondence, check grammar, punctuation, sentence length, agreement of subjects and verbs, and all other grammatical fine points

Although some ignore good writing skills in electronic correspondence, these guidelines are equally important whether you use paper or e-mail to transmit your message.

ANNOUNCEMENTS

Memos announcing employees joining your staff, job promotions, and other related events are conveyed with several characteristics in common. Sporting a complimentary tone, the memo should briefly present appropriate facts and information and state action steps, if any. An announcement memo should include the following:

- Event (eg, new staff member, position filled, promotions), including the name, position title, effective date, and line of reporting
- Responsibilities of new position
- Previous accomplishments
- Educational achievements
- Positive expectation
- Congratulations

NEWS

Internal memoranda are used for conveying good news and bad news, which may be a matter of perspective. When writing about a topic that may be disappointing to the reader (eg, budgetary cutbacks, disciplinary actions, documentation of discussion), use a neutral tone that just states the facts. Explain the reason for the communication. If there is a positive side, mention it. End the communication with an expression of goodwill.

MEETING NOTIFICATIONS

In addition to the date, place, and time, a memo announcing a meeting should have sufficient details to let the reader know the purpose of the meeting, to allow the reader to prepare for the event, and the reader should know what to expect as a result of the outcome of the meeting. If applicable, an agenda should be attached. The well-written notification would include the following information:

- Introduction or purpose (who, why)
- Details (what, when, and where)
- Preparation requirements (what to bring to or do before the meeting)
- Outcomes (what you are intending to achieve)

Close with a brief reaffirmation of the date, time, etc, expressed with goodwill.

Notification of training, workshops, and working meetings should be handled similarly but also may include:

- Purpose and benefits of attending
- Request for confirming attendance

The objective in writing these memos with all the necessary information included is to anticipate possible questions that will arise from the reader and address them. This time well spent avoids confusion and eliminates the need for further explanation. Figure 7-1 is an example of a meeting notification.

POLICIES

Writing good policy memos requires attention to detail because it usually means a change in behavior, at least for some readers. As Figure 7-2 illustrates, the ideal memo stating a new policy will include the following:

- State the new policy and the effective date
- Use a positive tone, particularly if the policy may not be received well or if it conveys bad news

- Offer a contact person who can give additional information or answer questions
- Close by conveying appreciation for following the policy

A memo that issues a change in policy requires notification of what change has occurred, anticipates questions that may arise from the policy change, and lets the reader know who is affected by the change. It should also provide a resource person for questions that may arise. Use clear, simple language when writing policies or memos that relate to them.

REQUESTS

Memos that request information or something of others must be clear, explain your rationale or need, and express appreciation to the reader. Ideally, the communication will include the following:

- Introduction or background (why)
- Clear request (what)
- Details (when do you need the information; where or how you want to receive it)
- Reason you are making the request (why)
- Thank your reader for the effort he or she will make on your behalf

RESPONSES

When you receive a written request, you should respond likewise, whether you agree or refuse the request. The ideal memo will have these components:

- Acknowledgment
- Agreement or refusal
- Reasons and explanation
- Tell what action you will take
- Express confidence in the outcome

Out of courtesy and respect, it is important not to overlook or ignore any point, being sure you respond to each issue.

REMINDERS

Reminders require certain details and always tact, as often they sound sharp rather than diplomatic. Since you are trying to get the reader to take action, you should keep in mind the following points when drafting your memos:

- Give specific details, such as dates, time, and location, as applicable
- Offer options, if available
- Express appreciation for the reader's cooperation
- Offer a resource for questions or assistance

CONCLUSION

Memorandums are internal documents used in medical practices for a variety of reasons and in many different ways. This style of communication is not intended for communicating with patients or for patient educational purposes. Although the format can be individualized and the method of transmittal may be mostly conveyed as an electronic version rather than a paper document, the content must be deliberate and consistent with the purpose intended. Although the "rules" are more informal than in external practice documents, such as correspondence and patient education papers, they should be carefully written to avoid confusion and misunderstanding by the reader. The way that you address your practice staff, in writing, can be very beneficial to achieving harmony and cooperation in your practice. Likewise, poorly written memos can be very detrimental to achieving your goals.

Effective Patient Communications

Medical practices use many forms and provide various patient education materials and instruction sheets as a part of their communications with patients. Each tool or document must be written with one goal in mind, that is, effective communication with the patient that gets the job done. Forms are used for gathering information or obtaining consent, and instructional documents are written to disseminate information. In both cases, the objective is *to get* or *to give* accurate information so that you can provide appropriate health care to the patient. After all, if your patient does not know what you are asking him or her to do, you are unlikely to achieve compliance with your care.

The purpose of this chapter is to provide some examples and explain some reasoning for presenting information in certain ways. You will do well to consider these aspects of communication a part of your strategy to manage risk in your practice, because you may be using poorly written documents where you are exposed to malpractice through professional negligence.

Some general guidelines should always be followed for patient education materials, such as the following:

- Name of the practice
- Name of the providers and their professional designations (eg, MD, DO, PA, NP, PT, OT)
- Address of the practice, including telephone number and fax
- Web site and e-mail information, if applicable
- Date the material was drafted

The practice's letterhead will take care of most of these prerequisites.

Likewise, the forms your practice uses should have the same identifiers. One of the most useful items to add to the forms that you develop is the date they were drafted. That way, you can always tell if the form you pick up is your most current revision or one that has surfaced long after it was replaced.

Refer to and use all the skills of good writing that are provided in prior chapters of this book, particularly Chapter 2.

The examples in this chapter are written to demonstrate readability, not to convey policy. The intent is for you to develop your own materials with content and style that reflect your protocols and practice.

INFORMATION

You will be continually issuing information to your patients in your role as a health care educator. But whether your patients are able to follow your thoughts and understand what you want them to know—or do— will depend on many factors. For example, Medicare can be confusing to anyone, particularly to those who are eligible to receive it. The letter in Figure 8-1 conveys to patients information regarding Medicare physicals. Figure 8-1 demonstrates how to inform an age group that may find it difficult to understand its payment responsibilities because of the complex nature of the payer. Whatever the demographics of your practice, you should write simply and clearly.

CONSENT

Informed consent is a process, not a form. For informed consent to be legally valid, physicians rendering the treatment or performing the procedure must afford patients who have the capacity sufficient information with which to make a decision about treatment. Whether sufficient or adequate information has been disclosed is a question of fact determined by differing standards. To determine what is required for informed consent, physicians must be aware of the law in their particular state.

Again, informed consent is a process, not a form. Forms serve mainly to document the process and comply with state law. A well-designed form coupled with a detailed physician's note in the medical chart may be the best evidence that the informed consent process took place.[1]

Figure 8-2 is provided for your review, but to use it you must adapt it to your state's law. Check with your local or state medical society for information regarding your state's requirements for obtaining informed consent. For surgical procedures, it is best to use a separate form and discussion process for use of anesthesia.

Some instances require you to inform the patient and to obtain written consent. For example, a dermatology practice may take photos of moles before and after treatment. Consent for imaging is such an instance (see Figure 8-3).

REMINDERS

You may have some form of system in place to remind your patients to schedule checkups or examinations, such as a diabetes checkup or a breast examination. A preprinted postcard that your patient addresses to himself/herself at the prior office visit is a good way to keep up with preparing this notice. You may wish your postcard format to resemble Figure 8-4.

OTHER EXAMPLES

You may develop handouts or send letters to your patients that will help them live with healthy habits or to explain some specifics of your practice style. The format you choose will most likely depend on the

F I G U R E 8 - 1

Sample Information Document

ABC Physician Group

1234 Wellness Blvd, Suite 56
Hometown, YZ 12345
555 666-7890
WWW.ABCGROUP.COM

Information Regarding Medicare Physicals

In our commitment to quality health care, the physicians of this practice regard annual physicals as a valuable tool to evaluate health maintenance. Nevertheless, Medicare does not pay for preventive medicine (eg, physical exams, certain laboratory tests, etc), even if you have a diagnosis.

The following explanation is presented to help you understand your charges:
When a patient comes in for an annual physician visit, we charge for an **office visit** for the discussion of ongoing **diagnoses**, and we charge for a **physical** for preventive **well care**. With our Medicare patients, we subtract the charges for the **diagnostic exam** and bill these charges to Medicare. The patient is responsible for the remaining portion of the **well care exam** at the time of the visit. This billing procedure follows Medicare guidelines and aids you in receiving the most coverage for your visit.

For example:

Well Care Exam	$350.00*
Diagnostic Exam	– 85.00 (to be filed with Medicare)*
Collectable from patient at visit	**$165.00**

* These figures are for example only and may not represent actual charges.

We submit the **diagnostic portion** of your exam to Medicare. On these visits only, we will accept assignment and file your secondary insurance for you. You may also receive additional well care procedures that Medicare does not cover, as explained in the Medicare waiver you sign. Any portion of the diagnostic exam remaining is your responsibility.

Although you will see two charges, this Medicare billing procedure is necessary for you to receive the best reimbursement your diagnosis will allow.

We hope this helps you understand your charges, and as always, our priority is providing the best quality health care for our patients. If you have any questions, please contact our billing office at 555 666-7890.

Issued 09/01/2004

FIGURE 8-2

Sample Patient Informed Consent Form

ABC Physician Group

1234 Wellness Blvd, Suite 56
Hometown, YZ 12345
555 666-7890
WWW.ABCGROUP.COM

Patient (or Authorized Representative's) Consent to Medical Treatment

I hereby give my consent for the performance of the following:
[insert name of procedure]

My physician has provided me with a general explanation of the nature of this treatment or procedure and the reasons for its indication for my particular medical condition.

My physician has also discussed with me the risks and benefits of the treatment. Some of these risks include, but are not limited to, the following:
[describe risks and benefits]

My physician has also explained that I can expect the following consequences and complications as a natural result of undergoing this intervention (some of which are attendant to any invasive procedure), although some of these may not occur, including but not limited to, the following:
[describe consequences and/or complications]

My physician has explained alternatives to undergoing this treatment or procedure, including:
[describe alternatives]

My physician has also explained the risks and benefits of forgoing the treatment or procedure recommended, including:
[describe risks and benefits of forgoing treatment]

My physician has also explained to me that other physicians and health care personnel will participate in my care.
[Physicians should insert a description here of the practice arrangement. For example, if residents are participating, explain, or if in group practice and another physician may substitute, disclose fully.]

I extend this authorization to these other physicians and health care personnel. Although unlikely, in the event that my physician is not available to perform the above treatment or procedure, I understand that this authorization may be extended to them. If possible, however, I will be notified of the substitution.

FIGURE **8-2**

Sample Patient Informed Consent Form—Continued

I also understand that during the procedure it may be necessary to administer other medical treatment. While I authorize necessary medical care, I limit this consent, however, to what is indeed medically necessary.

After discussing all of the above, my physician gave me an opportunity to ask questions and seek further information regarding the above items. I believe that I do not require further information at this time, and I am prepared to proceed with the recommended treatment or procedure. I believe that my physician has honored my right to make my own informed health care decision, give my consent voluntarily and freely, and certify that I can give valid consent (that is, I am not a minor or incompetent to make my own health care decisions). I understand that I can revoke this consent at any time up until the time that the treatment or procedure is started.

Patient's Printed Name: _____

Signature of Patient: _____

Time: _____ Date: _____

If the signature is of an authorized representative, the authorized representative is to complete and certify that the following is true: I am legally authorized to provide consent on behalf of the patient listed above. My relationship to the patient is described as follows:

Signature of Authorized Representative: _____

Signature of Witness [preferably family member]: _____

Relationship to Patient: _____

Issued 09/01/2004

ABC Physician Group

Source: Kinderman KL. *Medicolegal Forms With Legal Analysis: Documenting Issues in the Patient-Physician Relationship.* Chicago, Ill: American Medical Association; 1999:124-125.

FIGURE 8-3

Sample Information and Consent

ABC Physician Group

1234 Wellness Blvd, Suite 56
Hometown, YZ 12345
555 666-7890
WWW.ABCGROUP.COM

Consent for Imaging

I, [patient's name], understand that photographs, videotapes, digital, or other images may be recorded to document my care, and I grant consent to this.

I understand that ABC Physician Group will retain the ownership rights to these photographs, videotapes, digital, or other images but that I will be allowed access to view them or obtain copies of them, like any other portion of my medical record.

I understand that these images will be stored in a secure manner that will protect my privacy and that they will be kept for the time period required by law as outlined in ABC Physician Group's policy. Images that identify me will be released and/or used outside the institution only upon written authorization from me or my legal representative.

Patient's or Authorized Representative's printed name: _____

Patient's or Authorized Representative's signature: _____

Relationship to patient if other than self: _____

Witness: _____

Witness's signature: _____

Date and time: _____

Issued 09/01/2004

Source: Kinderman KL. *Medicolegal Forms With Legal Analysis: Documenting Issues in the Patient-Physician Relationship.* Chicago, Ill: American Medical Association; 1999:98.

F I G U R E 8 - 4

Sample Reminder Card

ABC Physician Group

1234 Wellness Blvd, Suite 56
Hometown, YZ 12345
555 666-7890
WWW.ABCGROUP.COM

It's that time again! Dr [name] would like to see you for your [6-month/annual/regular] [type of checkup or exam] around [_____].

Please call the office as soon as possible to schedule your appointment. Our schedule fills up quickly and we want to be able to accommodate you.

Issued 9/1/2004

seriousness of the message. For example, you may want to address all your senior patients with a generic handout. On the other hand, you may want to write a letter to your patients to explain a specific subject that is confusing to them. In this case, you will want your signature on the letter, as illustrated in Figure 8-5. An example of a generic form is provided in Figure 8-6.

CONCLUSION

When writing your patient education materials and even when drafting forms to gather information, you must consider these exercises as a part of your risk-management strategy. Outbound information must be clear and simply stated to get the best response from your readers. Forms that solicit inbound information should also be easy to understand so that you get accurate information from the one who is providing the answers. Remember to be guarded in what you say and how it is stated, and consider your tone. Putting a lot of effort into development of these communiqués will increase your level of patient compliance and will provide you with valid information on which to make your decisions for care.

ENDNOTE

1 Kinderman KL. *Medicolegal Forms With Legal Analysis: Documenting Issues in the Patient-Physician Relationship*. Chicago, Ill: American Medical Association; 1999:111.

FIGURE 8-5

Sample Patient Information Letter

Explanation of Fees

Dear Patient:

Your fee is based on the time I spend with you during your visit, the complexity of your medical condition, and the treatment you receive. Proper care for your health also requires that I, and others on my staff, spend time in activities other than your office visit or treatment time. This time may be used to:

- Create and maintain your permanent medical record
- Review, interpret, and document your laboratory work and tests and communicate those results to you by phone or by mail
- Review your current X rays or scan reports, compare them with prior reports, and, when studies are abnormal, consult with the radiologist
- Prepare and mail consultation reports and letters about follow-up visits to referring physicians
- Consult by phone with referring or consulting physicians and other health care providers
- Conduct phone calls with you and your family members for various reasons
- Send referral letters to additional specialists
- Distribute patient educational materials and medication samples when available
- Conduct medical research for your case through medical libraries or Internet search services
- Provide staff for your visit
- Arrange and coordinate other tests and consultations
- Communicate with pharmacies about your prescriptions
- Complete insurance applications and claim forms
- File insurance reports (eg, health claims, disability claims to insurance and state, Medicare disability)
- Conduct and negotiate utilization reviews with hospitals and insurance companies
- Review and manage hospital records
- Write letters of necessity to obtain medical services, instruments, or prescriptions for you
- Arrange for hospital admissions, house staff physicians, consulting physicians, and test and treatment facilities
- Communicate daily during admission with nurses, house staff, and attending physicians
- Complete tumor registry and other required reports
- Write orders for home health care and nursing facilities
- Provide reports and forms for various requests (eg, jury duty, school, job, sick leave, back to work, communicable disease)
- Participate in continuing medical education, clinical research, teaching, and medical writing to keep up-to-date on the latest medical advances

Although the cost of providing these services is high and always increasing, our practice is committed to keeping your costs low. We charge only what is necessary to provide you the highest standard of care. We look forward to a lasting and healthy relationship with you as our patient.

Sincerely,

Adapted from *Medical Practice Forms: Every Form You Need to Succeed,* by Keith Borglum and Diane M. Cate. ©2003. Published and distributed by PMIC, Los Angeles.

F I G U R E   8 - 6
Sample Patient Education Document

Health Care Advice for Seniors

Drive only as long as you are a safe driver.
Knowing when it's time to stop driving is important for your own safety and the safety of everyone on the road. I'll be happy to help you make the decision about when to give up your car keys; chronological age alone does not determine your fitness to drive.

Accept the aging process and its appearance.
Do you refuse to wear a hearing aid, eyeglasses, or dentures? Are you unwilling to ask for help or use walking aids? This behavior may make you accident-prone and prevent you from enjoying daily activities.

Discuss your health problems with me.
I can help you with many things that may be hard for you to discuss, such as sexual or urinary difficulties. Also, problems that you think are trivial—like stomach upsets, constipation, or jaw pain—may require further evaluation. Let me know what is bothering you so that I can help.

Ask me to repeat what I've told you about a health problem or treatment plan.
If you need more explanation or if you need for me to repeat what I have told you to do, ask me again. You can experience some serious health consequences unless you understand the information that I have given you.

Keep in mind the potential for a fall.
Falls result in fractures and painful injuries that may take months to heal. The following precautions will help guard against falling:

- Remove scatter rugs from your home.
- Make sure that your home and work areas are well lit.
- Wear sturdy, well-fitting shoes.
- Watch for slopes and cracks in sidewalks.
- Exercise to improve muscle tone and strength.

Have a system for managing medicines.
By using daily schedules, pillbox reminders, or check-off records, you can ensure that you take your proper medication doses. Because I and your other health care providers need to know all of the medicines you are taking, be sure to maintain a complete list of your prescription and over-the-counter medicines, including dose and the reason you are taking the medicine.

—Continued

FIGURE 8-6

Sample Patient Education Document—Continued

Have a single primary care physician.

By having a single primary care physician to monitor your health and evaluate treatment regimens, you can avoid the risk of being overtreated or undertreated.

Seek medical attention promptly.

Treatment delays, which may be due to denial, lack of money, or sense of inevitability, can result in a more severe illness and poorer prognosis. For this reason, get medical attention promptly for illness or injury.

Participate in prevention programs.

"An ounce of prevention is worth a pound of cure," so goes the old adage. To remain healthy, take advantage of readily available preventive health measures, such as flu and pneumonia shots, as well as routine breast and prostate exams.

Ask loved ones for help.

Alert family members to any signs of ill health. Getting the help you need may help you maintain your independence longer.

Adapted from Institute for Healthcare Advancement. Clip and Copy: Toward better senior healthcare: a handout to help older patients cope with the challenges of aging. *Medical Economics.* January 23, 2004.

Appropriate E-mail Use

Most new technologies take a while to settle in before people decide how to use them in the environment in which they work. E-mail is no exception to this rule. The norm in most medical practices is that e-mail is slow to catch on in spite of the convenience and opportunities this mode of communication offers. Nevertheless, physicians and their medical staffs in their homes and private lives may be avid users of computers and the Internet.

Why, then, are medical practices behind in the integration of e-mail into the practice environment? Perhaps there are several good reasons. The first may be a matter of work flow and the equipment available. It is also true that, by nature, interaction with patients is face-to-face, ear-to-ear, and hands-on, where verbal and visual messages tell a great deal more than words in electronic format could ever convey. Second, in the past, few practice workers have had the opportunity to sit all day at a computer or work station, as is common in other businesses. The most significant of the many reasons why physicians may be slow to adopt the use of e-mail in their practices is the concern over patient privacy and medical liability.

The issue of whether to use e-mail in your practice or in your personal and business matters will not be the main topic of this chapter. The discussion will be on how to use e-mail correctly and effectively if, and when, the decision is made to use it at all. Following is information every e-mail user needs to know about using e-mail at the professional level.

FORM

Correct form for e-mail has evolved into something very similar to the classic memo format as described in Chapter 7. Thus, you do not need to type salutations, such as "Dear [Name]" when starting your message because the e-mail is addressed to them in the first place. E-mail, by its predetermined format, starts with lines for designation of *to, from, copies,* and *subject.* Subject lines should define the topic and should be chosen carefully. Of course, you may choose to start out in a friendly way with a "Hello," "Good Morning," or similar greeting, although it is not necessary as a matter of form.

E-mail should be written properly using good grammar and correct spelling. In spite of its fast and casual nature, grammar, syntax, usage, and spelling should not be ignored. As with letters and other correspondence, the words you write and the way they are used are a reflection of your authority and credibility. All too often, writers get in a hurry and fail to read over what they have written and correct errors. Don't let the speed of e-mail foster sloppiness in your communication.

By design, e-mail is meant for brief messages. If your message is more than two paragraphs, consider using the telephone to convey your message.

ETIQUETTE

E-mail is almost like talking. We use it so much that we don't really think about it. But there are rules and courtesies that apply, just as there are with talking. And there are other considerations involved in communicating by written word only.

Most experts recommend avoiding e-mailing about emotional topics. Do not report bad news via e-mail. Don't fire someone or resign from a job via e-mail. Subjects of a serious nature should be handled in person unless it is simply not possible; in that case, use the telephone to conduct discussions or a business letter when documentation is needed.

The speed of e-mail fosters two other tendencies as well. One is rudeness (or abruptness); the other is the expectation that writers will hear back instantly from the correspondent. That prospect may not be realistic, particularly in medical practice, where the days are busy and the hours and minutes are filled with patient encounters, paperwork, telephone calls, and myriad interruptions.

If you use e-mail in your practice, be sure that you give your patients your policy on response time so that expectations are realistic for when they can expect a reply. Twenty-four to 48 hours is not unreasonable.

When you are writing e-mails, you may want to follow up on important items by making a phone call to ensure that your message gets through. Some e-mails never arrive at their intended cyber-destination. The prevalence of spam (which includes ads, jokes, and political petitions) is overwhelming in many instances. With spam filters in widespread use, be aware that some of your e-mail messages may not get through.

Other "dangers" of e-mail occur when emotions escalate and people send progressively angrier e-mails to one another, often saying things they regret. Remember that by writing in ALL CAPS and by using red type you can inflame someone, so avoid that as a measure of e-mail etiquette.

FUNCTION

More and more patients are choosing to e-mail their physicians. Access to their physicians rates high on the list of importance in the patient-physician relationship. Rather than waiting on hold or playing phone tag with their physicians, patients can ask direct questions and receive speedier responses. Patients love e-mail because the response can be read at the patient's convenience.

Meanwhile, the physician must look for that elusive balance between accessibility, which is good medicine, and efficiency, which is good business.

For the busy practitioner, the prospect of being inundated with complicated e-mails that raise multiple medical issues is daunting; especially when they are not paid for their time spent responding to those messages. This problem is not unique to e-mail, however, since physicians don't get paid for phone calls either.

Depending on the specialty or the nature of the practice, some physicians may want to have a controlled volume of e-mail traffic by selectively handing out an e-mail address to patients with chronic conditions, such as diabetes and high blood pressure, which need regular monitoring.

Another use is to have patients outline their questions before coming in for a checkup. This way, the visit is faster and more efficient because when the patient comes in, the physician knows exactly why. Some patients e-mail questions that they would like to talk about but find it difficult to discuss sitting in the office.

E-mail can be used for very straightforward matters, such as requests for medication refills or lab results. The ideal e-mail between the physician and the patient will:

- Be brief and to the point
- Be returned within 24 to 48 hours
- Not contain any bad news
- Be well written (ie, proper grammar, usage, punctuation, and spelling)
- Follow a written protocol for the kind of messages that are appropriate for e-mail (eg, for appointments, medication refills, lab results, etc; not for emergencies)
- Use appropriate subject lines

Avoid making the following mistakes when communicating through e-mail:

- Employing sarcasm
- Writing while you are angry
- TYPING IN ALL UPPERCASE or in red, which are the equivalent of yelling
- Sending e-mail to the wrong person
- Forgetting the attachment
- Clicking "send" too fast

Figure 9-1 provides an example of e-mail dialogue between a patient and physician.

By rereading the text before you send your e-mail, you can catch the majority of your mistakes. Look at the address line to make sure that

F I G U R E   9 - 1

Patient-Physician E-mail

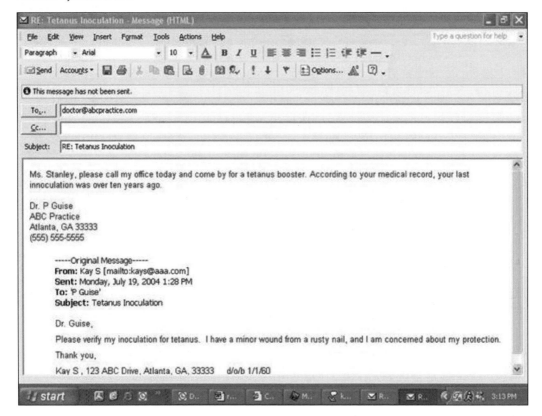

your subject line is not populated by a similar name rather than the intended addresses. Do not depend on the spell-checker entirely. It will catch misspellings but not incorrect word usage, such as *four* instead of *for* or *your* for *you're*. It also is unlikely to catch any missing words in a sentence that you inadvertently failed to include. So take a minute and reread your text before sending it.

PRIVACY

Privacy is an issue to address when using e-mail. Patient and physician exchanges should be sent through a secure system set up to protect the patient's privacy. Physicians can set up their own secure systems or subscribe to services, such as those set up by Medem, a communication network founded by a group of national medical associations. Patients who use such services pay a fee to e-mail their physicians.[1] Another secured service that is compliant with the Health Insurance Portability and Accountability Act (HIPAA) is MDhub (www.mdhub.com).

All e-mail exchanges should be deposited directly in the patient's medical record.

Under HIPAA, physicians have a responsibility to guard protected health information (PHI). In some cases, however, a patient may wish to have test results sent via e-mail and will sign a consent form for the communication. It is advisable to have the patient sign an authorization form to disclose PHI via e-mail. "The e-mail authorization should include language that clearly informs the patient that e-mail is not encrypted and the Internet is not secure. If the patient authorizes, it is permissible to send the results via e-mail," notes Laura Scallion, president and CEO of AllSource Technical Solutions, Inc, in Portland, Ore. Scallion advises entities to provide the form to the patient only upon request. A sample authorization form can be found in Figure 9-2.

The bottom line is this: You are permitted to send nonencrypted documents containing PHI to patients via e-mail as long as you first obtain a signed authorization from the patient explaining that transmissions sent over the Internet have vulnerabilities and are not 100% secure.[2]

INSTANT MESSAGING

Instant messaging (IM) is a cross between an e-mail and a phone call. It typically is used for very short notes and is not expected to be written in formal language, even in business or professional settings.

Pitfalls include messages popping up on your monitor unannounced. Messages appear automatically on the recipient's screen for anyone nearby to see. If you are on the phone or in a meeting, an instant message is an interruption. It is considered impolite to answer the IM while you are on a phone call or in a meeting. Etiquette experts recommend that you close your IM program or activate some sort of "busy" message before entering a meeting or taking a phone call.

Instant messages are just that, and it is possible to send multiple messages very rapidly. When composing an IM, send complete thoughts, even if in shorthand, and give the person a moment to respond. Many IM programs will inform you when your correspondent is typing a reply. Let them finish before responding again.

The ideal use of instant messaging includes the following:

- Compose your message in complete thoughts
- Allow the recipient a few moments to respond
- Do not send messages of a sensitive nature
- Close out your program when in a meeting or on a phone call
- Use proper grammar, punctuation, and spelling in all forms of electronic correspondence

Figure 9-3 illustrates an appropriate use of instant messaging functions within a practice.

Instant messaging is convenient, but it should be used with caution in a medical practice because of the proximity of your computer equipment to your patients.

FIGURE 9-2

E-mail Correspondence Authorization Form

Authorization for E-Mail Correspondence

Patient Name _____ Date of Birth _____ Medical Record Number _____

Verification of Identity (photo ID, if patient is unknown) _____ Social Security Number _____

**Complete the following only if the person completing the authorization is not the patient:

Name of Representative _____ Relationship to Patient _____ Legal Authority _____

Verification of Identity _____ Verification of Authority_____

By signing this form, I authorize: _____
(Person, class of person, or organization)

to communicate by electronic mail (e-mail) with me and with other health care providers as necessary for my/the patient's medical care and treatment.

I agree that e-mail messages may include protected health information about me/the patient, whenever necessary.

I understand that, by federal law, [Your Organization] may not use or disclose my health information, except provided in [Your Organization] Notice of Privacy Practices, without my authorization. My signature on this Authorization indicates that I am giving permission for the uses and disclosures of the protected health information described above. I hereby release [Your Organization] and its employees from any and all liability that may arise from the release of information as I have directed.

I understand that I have the right to revoke this Authorization at any time. If I want to revoke this Authorization, I must do so in writing, and address it to the person or institution named above. I understand that if I revoke this Authorization, it will not apply to any information already released as a result of this Authorization.

I understand that I may refuse to sign this Authorization; I also understand that the institutions or individuals named above cannot deny or refuse to provide treatment, payment, enrollment in a health plan or eligibility for benefits if I refuse to sign this Authorization.

I understand that, once information is disclosed pursuant to this Authorization, it is possible that it will no longer be protected by the federal medical privacy law and could be disclosed by the person or agency that receives it.

This Authorization expires automatically upon _____
Date or event

I have read and understand the information in this authorization form

Signature of Patient or Legal Representative: _____

Please print name: _____ Date:_____

FIGURE **9-3**

Physician-Staff Instant Message Communication

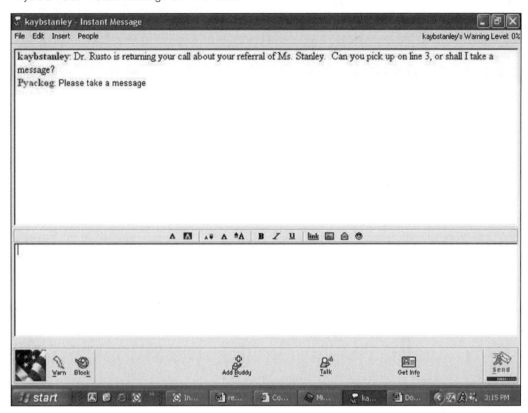

CONCLUSION

As the newest patient-physician conduit, e-mail can be a helpful tool for communicating with your patients and for interchanges with your staff and other business correspondence. The number of patients who send messages seeking medical advice or to make appointments is increasing steadily. Privacy, courtesy, accuracy, and professionalism are of utmost importance in all matters of correspondence, and e-mail and instant messaging are no exception. The medical practice that prepares in advance its standards and policies for use of e-mail will benefit most from its exchange with the patient and will be more satisfied with the results achieved.

ENDNOTES

1. Davidow J. The doctor will e-mail you now. *Seattle Post-Intelligencer*. Available at: http://seattlepi.nwsource.com/local/175159_hcenter27.html. Accessed May 27, 2004.
2. Eli Research Health Information Compliance Alert. The third degree: reader questions answered. *HIPAA on the Net*. 2004; 4, No. 2:14.

Tips for Letter-writing Ease and Proficiency

Writers often make mistakes expressing numbers in written documents, get confused over word choice of similar sounding words, and stumble over proper titles and abbreviations. The following lists may help you compose your letters quickly and accurately.

NUMBERS

- Spell out numbers at the beginning of a sentence.
- Spell out numbers from one through ten but use figures for numbers 11 and up.
- Use figures for fractions and units of measurement such as years (eg, 8 years) or page numbers (eg, page 7).

COMMONLY MISTAKEN WORDS

- *accept* "taking what is offered"
  except "meaning to exclude"
- *access* "available"
  excess "too much"
- *adapt* "change"
  adopt "making your own"
  adept "being skilled"
- *adverse* "unfavorable"
  averse "reluctant"
- *affect* "influencing"
  effect (noun) for "a result"
  effect (verb) "to bring about"
- *all ready* "readiness of multiples"
  already "something that previously happened"

- *allude* "an indirect reference (to)"
  elude "escaping (from)"
- *alumnus* "male graduate"
  alumna "female graduate"
- *biennial* "once every 2 years"
  biannual "twice a year"
- *ascent* "rising"
  assent "approval"
- *beside* "close to"
  besides "in addition (to)"
- *can* "physical ability"
  may "giving or requesting permission"
- *cession* "yielding"
  session "a meeting"

- *cite* "quoting"
  sight "seeing"
  site "a place to build a structure"
- *consul* "a government person"
  council "an assembly"
  counsel "advice"
- *decent* "suitable"
  descent "going down"
  dissent "disagreement"
- *disinterested* "impartial"
  uninterested "not interested"
- *forbear* "not doing something"
  forebear "ancestor"

- *ingenious* "skillful"
  ingenuous "candid"
- *precede* "coming before"
  proceed "going ahead"
  supersede "replacing"
- *statue* "sculpture"
  statute "a law"
- *their* "belonging to them"
  there "a place"
  they're "they are"
- *therefor* "for that"
  therefore "because of that"
- *waive* "giving up"
  wave "a swell of water"

NAMES AND TITLES

- Use *Mr.* or *Ms.* before a last name only if the person does not have a degree (eg, Mr. Love or Ms. Jones).
- Use a comma before Jr. (for junior) and Sr. (for senior) after a last name (eg, Peter Lewis, Sr.), but do not use a comma before a Roman numeral after a last name (eg, Norris Johns III).
- When someone has two or more academic degrees, arrange them after the person's name in this order: religious, theological, academic, and honorary.

ABBREVIATIONS FOR FORMS OF ADDRESS, TITLES, AND ACADEMIC DEGREES

Adj Adjutant
ADM Admiral
Asst Surg Assistant Surgeon
BA Bachelor of Arts
LLB Bachelor of Laws
BSN Bachelor of Science in Nursing
BG/Brig Gen Brigadier General
CPT/CAPT/Capt Captain
CPA Certified Public Accountant
COL/Col Colonel
CDR/Comdr Commander
CPL/Cpl Corporal
DDS Doctor of Dental Surgery
DD Doctor of Divinity
LLD Doctor of Laws
MD Doctor of Medicine
OD Doctor of Optometry

PharmD Doctor of Pharmacy
PhD Doctor of Philosophy
DPH Doctor of Public Health
DVM Doctor of Veterinary Medicine
1LT/1st Lt First Lieutenant
1SGT/1st Sgt First Sergeant
GEN/Gen General
Gov Governor
PharmG Graduate in Pharmacy
Lt Lieutenant
Lt Col Lieutenant Colonel
LCDR/Lt Comdr Lieutenant Commander
Lt Gen Lieutenant General
LTJG Lieutenant, Junior Grade
MAJ/Maj Major
MG/Maj Gen Major General

MS Master of Science or Master of Surgery
M Sgt Master Sergeant
PO Petty Officer
PA Physician Assistant
Pvt Private
PFC Private First Class
Prof Professor
RADM Rear Admiral
RN Registered Nurse

2LT/2nd Lt Second Lieutenant
SGT/Sgt Sergeant
SFC Sergeant First Class
SMA/Sgt Maj Sergeant Major
SSG/S Sgt Staff Sergeant
Supt Superintendent
Surg Surgeon
T Sgt Technical Sergeant
VADM Vice Admiral
WO Warrant Officer

RELIGIOUS SALUTATIONS

Roman Catholic
Dear Sister [name]:
Dear Reverend Mother:
Dear Father [name]:
Dear Monsignor [name]:
Dear Bishop [name]:
Dear Archbishop [name]:
Dear Cardinal [name]:
Your Holiness: (Only used when addressing the Pope.)

Protestant
Dear Mr. or Ms. or Dr. [name]:
Dear Reverend [name]:
Dear Bishop [name]:
Dear Archbishop [name]:

Jewish
Dear Rabbi [name]:

Islamic or Shiite
Your Eminence:

Sunni
Imam [name]:

Templates for Physician-related Employment Correspondences

Practice Opening for Associate

[date]

[inside address]

Dear Dr [name]:

Due to my large patient load, I am seeking a physician to assist with my busy [specialty] medical practice located in [city, state]. My first place to look for assistance is from my own alma mater, [name of institution].

I would appreciate it if you would post the enclosed notice where it can be seen by the senior [specialty] residents. When I receive responses, I will let you know.

Thank you for your assistance and please call me if you have questions.

Sincerely,

[name], MD

Enclosure

Practice Opportunity Form

Clinical specialist needed

[city, state of practice]

Start date: [date new physician is needed]
Date of posting: [date sent]

Board-eligible or board-certified [specialty] willing to join established solo [name of specialty] practitioner to share inpatient and outpatient care equally for [—] years, after which time [give terms]. Ability to perform [list procedures]. Pleasant demeanor and willingness to work an average of [—] hours a week. Excellent references and a [state] license are required.

Salary:
[$—] for year 1
[$—] for year 2, plus a bonus
[$—] for year 3, plus a bonus

Benefits:
[$—] professional liability insurance
[—] weeks of vacation a year
[$—] medical insurance for self and family
[—] weeks of sick leave a year
[—] weeks of continuing medical education, plus [$—] registration, travel, etc, a year
Cell phone and pager
Licenses, dues, etc..., up to [$—] a year
Full [%] shareholder in the corporation after [—] years of employment [with or without] buy-in

Contact: [name], MD
Office: [telephone number]
Home: [telephone number]
Beeper: [beeper number]
Fax: [fax number]

Response to Inquiry Regarding Practice Opening

[date]

[inside address]

Dear Dr. [name]:

I am currently completing my [—] year of residency in [specialty] at [—] in [city, state]. I would like to practice in your exact location. My personal special interests in medicine include [—].

The opportunity for me to practice in your area would be highly desirable. My curriculum vitae is enclosed.

Thank you for your time and attention. I look forward to hearing from you in the near future.

Sincerely,

[name], MD

Enclosure

Unsolicited Application Rejection: Negative Response

[date]

[inside address]

Dear Dr. [name]:

I received your letter and curriculum vitae. Unfortunately, I can offer you no encouragement regarding employment in this practice.

Best wishes for a successful search.

Sincerely,

[name], MD

Unsolicited Application Rejection: Positive Response

[date]

[inside address]

Dear Dr. [name]:

We received your inquiry regarding employment opportunities at [name of practice]. Currently, we do not anticipate any [specialty] openings for [—] years.

Your abilities are impressive, as are your accomplishments. You might wish to contact [name], MD, in [city, state]. [His/Her] number is [telephone number].

I appreciate your interest in [name of practice], and I wish you success.

Sincerely,

[name], MD

Invitation to Interview: Unstructured

[date]

[inside address]

Dear Dr. [name]:

Thank you for your letter. Your experience and accomplishments are commendable and I would like to meet you.

Can you visit sometime soon? Please call the office to set up an interview.

I look forward to hearing from you.

Sincerely,

[name], MD

Invitation to Interview: Structured

[date]

[inside address]

Dear Dr. [name]:

I am happy to tell you that I have been authorized to extend an invitation to you to visit [name of practice] the [—] week in [month]. I have enclosed a tentative itinerary for your review. If you have problems being relieved of your residency duties in [month], an alternative is the [—] week in [month].

I look forward to your visit.

If you have any questions or concerns, please call [name] at [telephone number].

Sincerely,

[name], MD

Postinterview Rejection: General

[date]

[inside address]

Dear Dr. [name]:

We have completed interviews of [—] candidates, including you.

The choice was difficult since all the candidates were well qualified. I regret that you were not selected but feel certain that you will find another fine practice without difficulty.

Thank you for the time you devoted to interviewing for our opening. It was a pleasure interacting with you.

Sincerely,

[name], MD

Postinterview Rejection: Specific

[date]

[inside address]

Dear Dr. [name]:

The selection committee convened on [date] to select the candidates who will become our medical associates in [month] of next year. Those selected are:

[name], MD [specialty], [residency]*

While you were not selected, you did interview very well and should have no difficulty finding the right spot.

Best wishes for your future from all of the physicians at [name of practice].

Sincerely,

[name], MD

*List all of those selected.

Past Employment and Training Reference Request

[date]

[inside address]

Dear Dr. [name]:

Dr. [name] has applied for a position as a staff physician with [name of facility] in [city, state]. [He/She] advised me that [he/she] worked with you for [—] years, ending [date]. If you will kindly complete the brief questionnaire on the attached page, I would be most grateful. I appreciate your time.

Dr. [name]'s signed permission for you to release information to me is enclosed.

If there is any reason you would rather not complete the questionnaire, call me collect at [telephone number] and we will have a confidential talk.

Sincerely,

[name], MD

Enclosure

Confidential Reference Form

RE: [name], MD

Dates employed or dates of training: _____

Eligible for rehire or advanced training: _____

Quality of work: _____

Quantity of work: _____

Interaction with staff:	❏ Excellent	❏ Average	❏ Below average
Interaction with patients:	❏ Excellent	❏ Average	❏ Below average
Interaction with physicians:	❏ Excellent	❏ Average	❏ Below average
Interaction with hospital personnel:	❏ Excellent	❏ Average	❏ Below average
Interaction with hospital administrator:	❏ Excellent	❏ Average	❏ Below average
Ethical behavior:	❏ Excellent	❏ Average	❏ Below average
Attendance:	❏ Excellent	❏ Average	❏ Below average

Additional comments:_____

_____

_____

_____   _____

Signature   Date

Past Employment Disclosure Authorization

I, [name], authorize [name of professor or former associate, name of training program and institution, or name of former practice] to answer any and all questions written or oral posed by [name of recruiting physician or name of recruiting practice] regarding my [employment or training] at [name of former practice].

_____   _____

[name of applicant], MD   Date

_____   _____

Witness   Date

Offer of Employment

[date]

[inside address]

Dear Dr. [name]:

I am pleased to confirm our offer of employment with [name of practice] at an initial yearly salary of [$—], effective [date].

We are very happy with our decision and hope that you feel the same. Your training and experience will blend nicely with the practice.

Our attorney is drafting the final employment contract, which contains all of the changes you requested. It will be mailed to you directly from [name of attorney]'s office.

Welcome to the team. I look forward to working with you.

Sincerely,

[name], MD

Introduction to Staff

Memorandum

DATE: [date]
TO: All staff
FROM: [name], MD
RE: Newly hired physician

We have been interviewing physician candidates for the last [—] [days/weeks/months]. I want to thank you, once again, for all that you contributed to the process. I also want you to be among the first to know who has been selected.

On [date], [name of hired physician], MD, will begin working with us. While all the candidates were excellent, I feel that you and I will work best with Dr. [name of hired physician]. Dr. [name of hired physician]'s curriculum vitae is attached for your review. Please look it over.

[He/She] will arrive in town about [date] and attempt to be settled by [date]. [He/She] will reside at [address]. Please be as helpful as possible with [his/her] relocation both in and out of the office.

[Name] will act as Dr. [name of hired physician]'s [assistant/nurse] temporarily. I expect that both [he/she] and Dr. [name of hired physician] will let me know when [his/her] patient volume is such that we should hire an additional [assistant/nurse] for [him/her] on a permanent basis.

[Name] will schedule [his/her] appointments. Please also attend to [his/her] pager and cell telephone.

[—] will be [his/her] day off. Our call schedule will be [give schedule]. However, Dr. [name of hired physician] will not begin call until [date].

[Name], please review coding with Dr. [name of hired physician] and make sure [he/she] is up to par with our compliance standards.

[Name] will handle all physician number and hospital privilege issues and guide Dr. [name of hired physician] through the orientation process. Dr. [name of hired physician] already has [his/her] state license. [Name], please make a list of everything I have neglected to mention and bring it to my attention.

Let's make Dr. [name of hired physician] feel welcome, needed, and quickly productive. I know you will like working with [him/her] and so will our patients.

Attachment

Introduction Letter for a New Associate

[date]

[inside address]

Dear Dr. [name]:

On behalf of [name of practice], I am happy to announce that, effective [date], Dr. [name] will be joining our staff in the specialty of [name of specialty]. Dr. [name] will begin seeing patients on that date.

A graduate of [college or university] with a [degree] in [subject], Dr. Brown received his doctorate from [medical school], where he graduated with honors. He completed his residency program in [name of specialty] at [name of institution]. Most recently, he has practiced in [name of city] since completing his training.

Our practice will be greatly enhanced with the addition of Dr. Brown. Dr. Brown will be calling you in the next few weeks to introduce himself and to schedule a time to meet with you. I know you will like [name] and will help make him feel welcome as soon as you meet him. Thank you in advance for this kindness.

Sincerely,

[name], MD

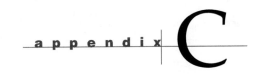
Templates for Staff-related Employment Correspondences

Offer of Employment

[date]

[inside address]

Dear [name of applicant]:

This letter will serve as follow-up to our telephone conversation and as confirmation of our offer to employ you in the position of [name of position] at [$—] an hour, effective [date], your first day of employment.

Although benefits were briefly described at the time of your interview, we will go over the benefits again with you on [first date of employment]. We'll also review our policies and answer any questions you may have prior to introducing you to our staff and physicians.

Thank you for accepting employment with us and welcome to [name of practice].

Sincerely,

[name]

Prior Employment Verification

[date]

[inside address]

To Whom It May Concern:

[Name of practice] is considering hiring [name of applicant] for the position of [name of position] pending verification of prior employment with you.

Enclosed is a signed statement from [name of applicant] authorizing this inquiry and a form for your response. Your candid replies will be held in the strictest confidence.

Please answer the few questions, make a copy for your files, and return the original to me in the enclosed preaddressed stamped envelope. Thank you for your kind assistance.

Sincerely,

[name]

Enclosures

Response Form

Name: [name of applicant]

Address: [—]

Starting date: _____

Departure date: _____

Position(s) held: _____

Would you rehire applicant?   ❑ Yes ❑ No

Did applicant give adequate notice of departure?   ❑ Yes ❑ No

Applicant's evaluations were generally:

     ❑ Excellent   ❑ Average   ❑ Below average

_____
Signature

_____
Name and title (print)

_____
Date

Reference Check

[date]

[inside address]

Dear [name]:

[name of applicant] has applied for a position with our medical practice and has identified you as a reference.

I realize that your time is valuable and, therefore, I am using the enclosed reply form to speed up the process.

Please answer the questions on the form and add anything you feel may be of value. Return the completed form in the preaddressed stamped envelope provided and return it to me as soon as possible.

If you prefer, you may fax the information to me at [fax number]. Please send with a cover sheet marked "confidential," if you choose to send your reference information by fax.

Thank you in advance for this information, which will help us process [name of applicant]'s application for employment with [name of practice].

Sincerely,

[name]

Enclosures

Reply Form

I have known this applicant for [—] years as a (check all that apply):
❑ friend   ❑ coworker   ❑ employee   ❑ patient   ❑ student   ❑ other

My opinion of [name of applicant] follows:

_____

Signature

_____

Name and title (print)

_____

Date

Notice to Staff Regarding New Hire

Memorandum

DATE: [date]
TO: All staff
FROM: [name]
RE: [name of applicant]

[Name of applicant] has been selected as our new [job title]. [He/She] will begin [his/her] employment and orientation on [date].

[name of applicant]'s education includes a [name of degree] from [name of institution] and certification from [name of certification agency]. [His/her] employment background includes [names and titles of recent relevant positions].

Please help me to welcome and make [name of applicant] feel like part of our team from [his/her] first day of work.

Orientation Introduction

[date]

[inside address]

Dear [name of applicant]:

The enclosed orientation plan will give you a good idea of what to expect during your first week with [name of practice]. Hopefully, being able to clearly anticipate what's ahead will ease any new job jitters you may have.

Our staff and physicians are eager to greet you on [first date of employment].

Your orientation plan is as follows:

Day 1: [date]
[——]*

Day 2: [date]
[——]*

Day 3: [date]
[——]*

Day 4: [date]
[——]*

Day 5: [date]
[——]*

Sincerely,

[name]

Enclosure

*List exact starting and ending times for all introductions, meetings, breaks, lunches, and any other pertinent information.

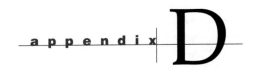

Templates for Human Resources-related Internal Practice Correspondences

Performance Appraisal: Improved

[date]*

[inside address]

Dear [name]:

It is my pleasure to document our discussion of your performance appraisal.

You have improved all prior performance deficits, specifically [describe problem area(s)]. I am encouraged with your turnaround and appreciate your efforts to improve. Keep up the good work.

Sincerely,

[name]

*This may also be in the form of a memorandum.

Performance Appraisal: Poor

Memorandum[*]

DATE: [date]
TO: [name]
FROM: [name]
RE: Performance

This memorandum will serve to document our discussion and meeting on [date] during which you were advised that your performance is below our acceptable standard. Specifically, you are deficient in the following areas:

[—][†]

I plan to receive reports from [name] weekly for the next [—] weeks. At the end of the [—]-week period, if little or no improvement is evident, I will have little choice other than to terminate your employment. You have been warned orally [—] times and this constitutes your [—] written warning.

I hope we can work together to help your performance improve.

[*]This may also be in the form of a letter.
[†]List all areas of unacceptable performance, such as the inability to interact with patients in a cordial manner, constant tardiness, or refusal to learn a computer system.

Probationary Period: Successful Completion

Memorandum[*]

DATE: [date]
TO: [name]
FROM: [name]
RE: Probationary period

Congratulations! Your probationary period ends today, and you are an exemplary member of our staff.

As we discussed prior to your employment, [—][†] will now be initiated.

[*]This may also be in the form of a letter.
[†]List any conditions that might now apply, such as full benefits or a raise.

Probationary Period: Unsuccessful Completion

[date]*

[inside address]

Dear [name]:

This letter is to inform you that your employment with this practice is hereby terminated. Working in a physician's office takes a special calling and is not a good fit for everyone. I wish you well as you seek a position where your talents might better be used.

Upon handing you this letter, please [—].† I will then [—].‡

Please contact [—] about health insurance and other termination issues.

Your final paycheck [—].§

Sincerely,

[name]

---

*This may also be in the form of a memorandum.
†List what the departing employee should do, such as remove all personal belongings or turn in keys.
‡List what employer or supervisor will do, such as escort departing employee out.
§State whether the final paycheck will be given to the employee now or sent later.

Probation Period: Unsuccessful Completion With Extension of Probation

[date]*

[inside address]

Dear [name]:

Your probationary period will end next week on [date].

You have made great progress and will undoubtedly continue to do so. However, you are not as far along in the completion of your training as expected. Therefore, I am extending your probation for an additional [—] days. This should give you enough time to complete the training plan and show an improvement.

If you have questions or concerns, please feel free to visit me.

Sincerely,

[name]

*This may also be in the form of a memorandum.

Disciplinary Action: Warning

Memorandum[*]

DATE: [date]
TO: [name]
FROM: [name]
RE: [subject of warning]

You have repeatedly [describe offense]. You have read and signed a statement that you have read our policies and understand them. However, [describe offense] continues, although our policies are clearly stated.

Please consider this warning as an official directive for corrective action on your part.

[*]This may also be in the form of a letter.

Disciplinary Action: Reprimand

[date][*]

[inside address]

Dear [name]:

This is a formal letter of reprimand.

On [date] you [describe offense] on the premises of [name of practice], which is strictly against our policy. Please take note of this reprimand and review our policies with particular attention to [—].

Thank you for your anticipated cooperation.

Sincerely,

[name]

---

*This may also be in the form of a memorandum.

Disciplinary Action: Suspension

[date]*

[inside address]

Dear [name]:

Disciplinary action is being taken against you in the form of a [—]-day suspension from work effective [date] and ending [date].

Disciplinary action is being taken based on the following facts: [describe offense]†

This [—]-day suspension without pay is considered formal disciplinary action. A record of this disciplinary action will be put in your personnel file.

If you wish to respond, please do so in writing by [date]. You may waive your right to respond by failing to do so prior to [same date as stated above].

It is of paramount importance that you reflect on your offensive actions during the suspension period. After the suspension period, it is expected that you will return ready to fully comply with our practice policies, rules, and regulations. Failure to do so will result in termination.

Sincerely,

[name]

---

*This may also be in the form of a memorandum.

†List the offense(s), such as asking someone to clock in for him or her or refusing to perform a duty.

Termination: Without Cause, Immediate

[date]

[inside address]

Dear [name]:

This letter is to inform you of the decision to terminate your employment immediately.

Upon handing you this letter, please [—].* I will then [—].†

Please contact [—] about health insurance and other termination issues.

Your final paycheck [—].‡

I hope you will be able to find new employment in the near future. Thank you for the time and effort you have put into this practice.

Sincerely,

[name]

*List what the departing employee should do, such as remove all personal belongings or turn in keys.
†List what the employer or supervisor will do, such as escort departing employee out.
‡State whether the final paycheck will be given to the employee now or sent later.

Termination: Without Cause, With Two Weeks' Notice

[date]

[inside address]

Dear [name]:

This letter will formalize your termination as of [date].

During the next 2 weeks, it is expected that you will complete your ongoing duties in a professional and satisfactory manner.

Please contact [—] about health insurance and other termination issues.

Your final paycheck [—].[*]

I hope you will be able to find new employment in the near future. Thank you for the time and effort you have put into this practice.

Sincerely,

[name]

[*]State whether the final paycheck will be given to the employee on the last day of employment or sent later.

Termination: Lack of Work or Downsizing

[date]

[inside address]

Dear [name]:

This is to inform you that your position is being eliminated as of [date]. I appreciate your [—] [months/years] of loyalty and excellent performance, and I will be happy to provide any reference you may need in the future.

Upon handing you this letter, please [—].[*] I will then [—].[†]

Please contact [name] about health insurance and other termination issues.

Your final paycheck [—].[‡]

Thank you for everything.

Sincerely,

[name], MD

---

[*]List what the departing employee should do, such as remove all personal belongings or turn in keys.
[†]List what employer or supervisor will do, such as escort departing employee out.
[‡]State whether the final paycheck will be given to the employee now or sent later.

Restructuring of Practice

Memorandum

DATE: [date]
TO: All staff
FROM: [names of all physicians in the practice]
RE: Restructuring

[Name of practice] has been sold to [name of purchaser] effective [date].

We will become employees of [name of purchaser] and, as of this time, each of us will remain with the practice. [Name of purchaser] [has/has not] agreed to retain all the current full-time and part-time employees.

Changes are certain to occur. Some we may like and some we may not. We ask your cooperation and positive demeanor during the transition.

Our main concern, as always, is the welfare of our patients. We can best serve them by making the transition appear as seamless as possible and by maintaining a caring attitude.

[Name of employee] has been appointed transition advocate. Please bring any concerns to [him/her].

Thank you for your great teamwork and your cooperation.

COBRA: Death of Employee

[date]

[inside address]

Dear [name of spouse of deceased employee]:

[Name of deceased employee]'s untimely death has our staff grieving with you. [Name of deceased employee] was an excellent employee and a delight to work with.

As [his/her] spouse, you and your minor children are entitled to continue in the practice group health insurance plan for [—] months. Your cost is based on a percentage that will total [$—] a month for the entire family. You became eligible for this coverage immediately on [name of deceased employee]'s death and your eligibility extends for [—] days from that date.

Please contact [—] about further information concerning keeping this coverage current. Please let me know as soon as possible how you wish to proceed on this matter.

My thoughts are with you and your family.

Sincerely,

[name]

COBRA: Divorce or Legal Separation

[date]

[inside address]

Dear [name of separated spouse or ex-spouse of employee]:

Under the Consolidated Omnibus Budget Reconciliation Act (COBRA), as the [divorced spouse/legally separated spouse] of [name of employee], you are eligible to receive health care benefits under our practice health insurance plan. You became eligible on the date of your [divorce/legal separation] and that eligibility extends for a total of [—] days. As of this writing, you have [—] days remaining to decide if you wish this coverage or not.

It will be necessary for you to remit a premium of [$—] to the practice each month in the amount of [$—]. This will ensure that coverage is not cancelled.

Please contact [—] about further information concerning keeping this coverage current. If we have not heard from you by [date], you will no longer be covered by [name of insurance company].

Sincerely,

[name]

COBRA: Employee With Medicare

[date]

[inside address]

Dear [name of spouse of employee]:

Since [name of employee]'s health insurance coverage will be through Medicare as of [date], I am writing to advise you of your rights under the Consolidated Omnibus Budget Reconciliation Act (COBRA).

You are eligible to continue benefits from our medical practice's health insurance coverage for [—] months after [name of employee] begins Medicare coverage. However, you must elect to continue with [name of practice]'s insurance within [—] days of the beginning of [name of employee]'s first Medicare coverage.

It will be necessary for you to remit a premium to the practice each month in the amount of [$—]. This will ensure that coverage is not cancelled.

Please contact [—] about continuing this coverage. If we have not heard from you by [date], you will no longer be covered by [name of insurance company].

Sincerely,

[name]

Response to Request for Payout of Pension Benefits After Termination

[date]

[inside address]

Dear [name of former employee]:

Here is information concerning your retirement plan payout.

At the time of your termination of employment, you were [—]% vested in the practice retirement plan because you had completed [—] full years of employment with [name of practice].

Each year the plan pays for a valuation of the plan assets and each participant is advised of his or her individual asset amount. Because you are asking for a separate valuation prior to the plan's regularly scheduled valuation at the end of the year, it will be necessary for the cost of this valuation to be taken out of your funds. If you wait until the end of the year, this fee will not be taken from your balance. I have contacted the plan's administrator and learned that the fee for this service will be [$—].

Please complete and return the enclosed election form along with instructions on the valuation date.

Sincerely,

[name]

Enclosure

Memorandum

DATE: [date]
TO: All staff
FROM: [name]
RE: Personnel policies

At the time of hire, every employee was given a handbook that briefly explained what to expect from the practice and what the practice expects from its employees. The handbook was based on our personnel policies adopted in [year].

As of [date], our personnel policies have been revised. Here is a copy of the revised policies. A revised copy of the handbook will be available by [date].

As of [date], the effective date of the new personnel policies, each staff member will be asked to sign and date a statement verifying that they have read and understand the new policies. Thank you for your cooperation.

Attachment

Unused Vacation

[date]

[inside address]

Dear [name]:

Our policy states that no more than [—] [hours/days] of vacation may be carried over from one [calendar year/employment year] to another.

According to our records, you have [—] vacation [hours/days] available, [—] of which you will lose if not taken before [date].

Please let us know what your intentions are concerning this issue by [date].

Sincerely,

[name]

Overutilization of Benefits

[date]

[inside address]

Dear [name]:

It has been brought to my attention by [name] that you have overutilized the benefits afforded you by the practice. Our records indicate that you have [—].*

Please review the above information for accuracy and contact [—] to make an appointment to resolve this issue.

Sincerely,

[name]

*Describe the type of overutilization of benefits, such as taken more vacation hours or days than accrued, taken more sick days than accrued, or used the resources of the physicians on staff more times than allowed.

Reference for Departing Employee: Favorable

[date]

[inside address]

Dear [name]:

[Name of departing employee] has asked that I write a letter of recommendation based on my knowledge of [his/her] work during [his/her] [—] years with [name of practice]. [Name] is [—].[*]

I feel very comfortable recommending [name of departing employee] as [his/her] record with [name of practice] is excellent.

Sincerely,

[name]

[*]Describe the positive traits or skills of the departing employee, such as being an enthusiastic worker or someone with great attention to detail.

Departing Employee: Verification of Dates of Service

[date]

[inside address]

Dear [name]:

This letter is to verify [name of departing employee]'s dates of service with us, which were [date] to [date].

Sincerely,

[name]

Confidentiality Agreement

Memorandum

DATE: [date]
TO: All staff
FROM: [name]
RE: Confidentiality agreement

Our medical practice has adopted the attached confidentiality agreement. All employees, both current and future, including all physicians, are required to sign and date this agreement with a witness present. The witness must also sign the confidentiality agreement. Please turn in your signed agreement by [—]. Thank you.

Attachment

Confidentiality Agreement Form

As an employee of [name of practice], I hereby certify that all knowledge or information I gain from [name of practice], whether trade secrets, expertise, technical data or information, transparencies, test data, or patient information revealed to me as strictly confidential, will be held in strict confidence and trust by me.

I will not reveal or disclose the trade secrets or information on patients or physicians to any other person, firm, corporation, company, or other entity now or in the future, unless my employer instructs me to do so. This secrecy protection will continue even if I no longer am employed by [name of practice]. I understand that if I reveal any of this confidential information to unauthorized persons, I personally may be subject to penalties and lawsuits for injunctive relief and money damages as well as possible criminal charges.

_____

Signature of employee

_____

Name of employee (print)

_____

Signature of witness

_____

Name of witness (print)

_____

Date

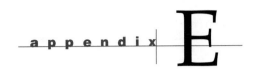

Templates for Other Human Resources-related Internal Practice Correspondences

Departing Physician

Memorandum

DATE: [date]
TO: All staff
FROM: [name]
RE: Dr. [name of departing physician]'s departure

[Day], [date], will be Dr. [name of departing physician]'s last day with [name of practice]. [He/She] plans to move to [city, state] where [he/she] will [—].[*]

Dr. [name of departing physician]'s patients will be sent an appropriate letter concerning [his/her] departure. We will ask Dr. [name of departing physician]'s patients to select a new physician from our group. After [date], please do not schedule any new patients for Dr. [name of departing physician].

I anticipate that each of you will make this transition as painless as possible for the patients. Thank you for your cooperation.

---

[*]State what departing physician plans to do, such as start a solo practice or join a teaching staff.

Sale of Practice

[date]

[inside address]

Dear [name]:

You, along with every other employee of [name of practice], are receiving this letter informing you of our unanimous decision to sell this practice to [name of purchaser]. The final sale closing date is [date]. After this date, we will all be employees of [name of purchaser].

We reached this decision with extensive analysis and forethought, concluding that a sale was the best move for you, for our patients, and for us. As time passes, we hope that you will agree that we made the right decision.

Thank you for your understanding and anticipated loyal cooperation during the transition.

Sincerely,

[name], MD*

---

*List names of all the physicians in the practice.

Practice Merger

Memorandum

DATE: [date]
TO: All staff
FROM: [names of all physicians in the practice]
RE: Practice merger

On [date], [name of practice] and [name of other practice] will officially merge. The name of the merged practice will be [—].

I anticipate that you may be somewhat anxious about your job security. Please don't be. We have [—] months to work out all of the details, and we will apprise you regularly so that you can know what to expect.

Thank you for your cooperation.

Congratulations: Promotion Within Practice

[date]

[inside address]

Dear [name]:

Congratulations on your promotion to [name of position]. This practice certainly benefits from your expertise and positive influence. We appreciate your contributions and are proud to have you with us.

Sincerely,

[name]

Congratulations: Outside Award or Recognition

[date]

[inside address]

Dear [name]:

Congratulations from all of us at [name of practice].

Your [name of award/recognition] is a great [accomplishment/achievement] and makes us doubly proud to have you as part of our practice team. Keep up the good work.

Sincerely,

[name]

Condolences

[date]

[inside address]

Dear [name]:

The people you work with daily are devastated over [name of deceased]'s death. There are no words to express our sympathy for the profound loss you have suffered.

Please know that we are thinking of you.

The physicians of [name of practice] will make a donation to [name of charity] to honor [name of deceased]'s memory.

Sincerely,

[name]

Change of Location

Memorandum

DATE: [date]
TO: All staff
FROM: [name]
RE: Relocation of our Practice

Our lease will expire on [date]. We have not been able to come to terms on a new lease at our present location. We have located another suitable medical suite just [—] [blocks/miles] from our current location. Our new address will be [—].

We will communicate the move to our patients by mail and by placing an announcement in the newspaper.

Our move date will be [day], [date]. To accommodate the move, we will plan to be closed from [date] to [date]; please do not schedule patients for this time. However, our physicians will see emergencies at the hospital.

The moving firm will pack everything to be moved on [—] at the end of the work day. We will not have access to this location after that time. If you have personal items or work-related items that are fragile, please move them yourself.

Our work day at the new location will begin on [date] at the usual time. All staff members are expected to report on time.

Thank you for your help and cooperation.

Opening a Satellite Office

Memorandum

DATE: [date]
TO: All staff
FROM: [name]
RE: New Satellite Office

In order to attract new patients, and also to take some of the strain off our present facility, we are opening a satellite office at [address]. Our anticipated opening date is [date].

Soon, we will decide our schedule for covering the medical care at this new location, and we will advise you of any changes shortly.

We will need [—]* at the satellite office. If you wish to transfer to the new location, please contact [—]. We will handle requests on a first-come, first-served basis.

Thank you.

*Describe the staff positions that will be needed, such as receptionists, nurses, medical assistants, and account representatives.

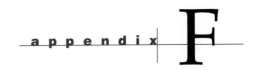

Templates for Patient-directed External Practice Correspondences

Welcome to New Patient

[date]

[inside address]

Dear [name]:

Thank you for scheduling an appointment with Dr [name] on [day], [date]. It is my pleasure to welcome you to [name of practice] in advance of your first visit.

The patient information enclosed will help familiarize you with the practice and how we operate. If you have any questions after reading the material, I will be happy to answer them for you by telephone prior to your visit. Also enclosed is a patient registration form. Please complete the form and either fax it to us at [fax number] or bring it with you to your appointment.

We appreciate your selecting Dr [name] for your medical care and will work hard to serve your needs.

Sincerely,

[name]

Enclosures

Response to Patient With a Complaint

[date]

[inside address]

Dear [name]:

I received your letter today and want you to know that I deeply regret your dissatisfaction with our office. Thank you for letting us know about [reason for complaint]*.

We will investigate the situation you described, and I will speak to you soon about the results. Meanwhile, please accept my apology for the unpleasant experience, and let me know if I can help you in any other way.

Sincerely,

[name]

*Describe the alleged reason for the complaint, such as a long wait time or an inconsiderate employee.

Condolences to Spouse on Death of Spouse

[date]

[inside address]

Dear [name]:

Over the last few [months/years], it has been our pleasure to assist a very special [man/woman]. Your [husband/wife] was just that, very special, which made it so easy for us to try to help [him/her].

It is difficult for us to imagine the depth of your loss, but we feel that we share the loss. We hope it gives you comfort to know that we will always remember [name of deceased] at [name of practice] in the kindest and most loving way.

Sincerely,

The staff of [name of practice]

Condolences to Parent on Death of Child

[date]

[inside address]

Dear [Mr/Ms] [name]:*

Loving a child the way we witnessed your love for your [son/daughter][name] must be one of the greatest gifts of parenting. We were privileged to have known [him/her] and share in the loss.

Please accept our sincere condolences, and know that you are in our hearts and thoughts at this time of sorrow.

Sincerely,

The staff of [name of practice]

*Address to both parents if they live in the same household.

Examination or Test Results: Normal/Negative

[date]

[inside address]

Dear [name]:

The results of your [—]* are [normal/negative]. A copy of this record is enclosed for your files.

Dr. [name] sends best wishes and thanks for allowing [him/her] to care for your medical needs.

Sincerely,

[name]

*Describe the type of results or findings that are normal/negative, such as x-rays or blood tests.

Examination or Test Results: Abnormal/Positive

[date]

[inside address]

Dear [name]:

The results of your [—]* are [abnormal/positive], and so I feel additional tests are indicated.

Please contact [name] for further information. I have given full instructions to [him/her] on the next steps to take. After you have spoken to [name], please call me with any other questions or concerns you may have.

Sincerely,

[name], MD

*Describe the type of results or findings that are abnormal/positive, such as x-rays or blood tests

Appointment Reminder Notice

[date]

[inside address]

Dear [name]:

It's that time again! Dr. [name] would like to see you for your [6-month/annual/regular] [—]*
around [—].†

Please call me as soon as possible to schedule your appointment. Our schedule fills up quickly, and
we want to be able to accommodate you.

Sincerely,

[name]

---

*State the type of checkup or examination, such as a diabetes checkup or a breast examination.
†Link the appointment to a familiar event or holiday, such as Labor Day or after the school year begins.

Patient Satisfaction

[date]

[inside address]

Dear [name]:

Once a year we feel it is necessary to examine our practice from our patients' point of view.

We have selected [—] patients to participate in an opinion survey. We try to select different people every year. You have been selected this year, and this letter is your invitation.

Please complete the enclosed survey and return it to us in the preaddressed stamped envelope provided. The entire process should take you only about 10 minutes. Your input will help us improve the practice for you and all our patients.

Sincerely,

[name], MD*

Enclosures

*List the names of all of the physicians in the practice.

Patient Satisfaction Survey

		True	False	N/A
Name of your physician: _____				
Please check (in the appropriate box) if the statement is true, false, or not applicable (N/A).				
1.	My physician acts like he/she cares about me.	☐	☐	☐
2.	My physician seems knowledgeable.	☐	☐	☐
3.	My physician answers my questions.	☐	☐	☐
4.	My physician explains everything clearly.	☐	☐	☐
5.	I have seen my physician only in the office.	☐	☐	☐
6.	I have seen my physician only in the hospital.	☐	☐	☐
7.	I have seen my physician in the office and in the hospital.	☐	☐	☐
8.	His/Her office hours are convenient.	☐	☐	☐
9.	I can get an appointment easily.	☐	☐	☐
10.	My insurance is always filed correctly.	☐	☐	☐
11.	The fees or co-payments are reasonable.	☐	☐	☐
12.	The staff is cordial and helpful.	☐	☐	☐
13.	There are sufficient parking spaces.	☐	☐	☐
14.	I have referred other patients to this practice.	☐	☐	☐
15.	The wait in the reception area is usually less than 20 minutes.	☐	☐	☐
16.	I would change physicians if my physician stopped participating in my insurance plan.	☐	☐	☐
17.	Other members of my family use this practice.	☐	☐	☐
18.	If my physician referred me to a specialist, I would go.	☐	☐	☐
19.	I appreciate the office decor and cleanliness.	☐	☐	☐

Payment Collection: Early Intervention

[date]

[inside address]

Dear [name]:

A review of unpaid accounts indicates that you have an overdue balance of [$—].

You may use the enclosed preaddressed stamped envelope to send us a check or to provide credit card information to pay off the outstanding balance. Or, as an alternative, call us at [telephone number] and give us your credit card information over the telephone in order to transfer your balance.

If you have any questions, please call me at [phone number/extension number] and I will be happy to discuss them. We value you as a patient.

Sincerely,

[name]

Enclosure

Payment Collection: Mid Intervention

[date]

[inside address]

Dear [name]:

You have an outstanding account balance of [$—] for medical services rendered by Dr. [name].

Your unpaid account is being considered for legal action. Once again, we urge that you mail your check today. Enclosed is a preaddressed stamped envelope for your convenience. If you wish instead, we will transfer your balance to a credit card of your choice.

If you are having financial problems, please let us hear from you. This will enable us to work with you on a mutually satisfactory financial solution. Although we value you as a patient, we cannot carry your account any longer without a response from you.

Sincerely,

[name]

Enclosure

Payment Collection: Nonresponse From Insurers (Letter to Patient)

[date]

[inside address]

Dear [name]:

It has been more than [—] months since we filed your insurance claim. However, your insurer has made no payment.

We contacted your insurance company for the status of your claim, yet to date, we have had no response from our inquiries. Our policy is to await payment from insurers for [—] days.

Although we have tried to collect payment from your insurance company, you will now have to pursue this matter with [name of insurance company].

Please mail us a check today for [$—]. A preaddressed stamped envelope is enclosed for your convenience. Or call us with credit card information and we can transfer the balance to the credit card of your choice.

Please call me at [telephone number] so that we may finalize this matter without delay.

Sincerely,

[name]

Enclosure

Payment Collection: Late Intervention

[date]

[inside address]

Dear [name]:

As a result of your nonresponse to our many requests for payment or communication, we are forced to take action.

Therefore, we have authorized [name of law firm] to do whatever is legally possible to satisfy the debt you incurred.

Sincerely,

[name]

Patient Financial Review Form

Name of patient _____

Balance due _____   Date of last patient visit _____

Reason for nonpayment or for lack of contact:

❏ Patient is deceased   ❏ Patient refused to pay

❏ Mail returned   ❏ Payment is late or not paid in ___ months

❏ Patient's telephone is disconnected or number changed

❏ Patient moved out of state

❏ Other: _____

Telephone contact: ❏ Yes   ❏ No

Dates of telephone contact: _____

Discussed a payment plan with patient: ❏ Yes ❏ No

Highlights of discussion:

_____

_____

Which collection letters were sent? _____

Have all payments from insurance company been received?   ❏ Yes   ❏ No

Amount outstanding _____   How old is bill? _____

Staff recommendation:

❏ Write off   ❏ Settle for partial payment   ❏ Send to collection

Physician's recommendation:

❏ Write off   ❏ Settle for partial payment   ❏ Send to collection

Terminate care?   ❏ Yes   ❏ No

_____   _____

Signature of physician   Date

This financial review form should be attached to the patient's chart along with an itemized statement of the account. Provide additional documentation, if necessary.

Patient Dismissal for Various Reasons

Termination of Care

Return Receipt Requested

[Date]

[Inside Address]

Dear [name]:

I find it necessary to inform you that I am withdrawing from providing medical care for (you/your children) effective [_____] (include a reasonable time period, based on the patient's condition and course of treatment, usually two to four weeks in the future). I will be available to provide treatment until that date should (you/your children) require medical attention.

I recommend that you continue (your/your children's) care with another physician within the next [_____] weeks so that you may continue your treatment for [_____]. If you are unable to find a facility, you can contact [_____] (list resources, such as county medical society and/or specialty board; list telephone numbers and Web site addresses). These organizations will be able to provide you with the names, addresses, and telephone numbers of several other physicians in the area.

In order to help the transition process, I will make your medical records available to you or a physician of your choice. After we receive a written release from you, we will send your treatment records to your new provider.

Sincerely,

[name], MD

Announcing a New Health Care Provider to Patients

[date]

[inside address]

Dear [name]:

It is a pleasure to introduce you to our new [—],[*] [name]. [Name] joined the practice [date] and is already a very welcome addition to our health care team.

[He/She] graduated from [name of college/university] and received [his/her] [—][†] from [name of school]. Although [name] is able to care for any medical condition, [his/her] specialty is [subject/disease].[‡] [He/She] also has a particular interest in [—].[§]

[Name] will be scheduled to see patients [day] through [day] from [—] o'clock to [—] o'clock.

Please share this good news with your family, friends, and neighbors.

Sincerely,

[name], MD

---

[*]State the type of health care provider who is being introduced, such as a nurse practitioner, physician's assistant, or physician.

[†]State the type of degree, such as nursing degree or doctorate.

[‡]State the type of care the new health care provider specializes in, such as obstetrics and gynecology or pediatrics.

[§]State the type of subject or disease the new health care provider is interested in, such as attention deficit disorder or epilepsy.

Opening a Satellite Office

[date]

[inside address]

Dear [name]:

You may have seen our recent announcement in the [name of newspaper] concerning the opening of our satellite office at [address]. Although the office officially opened on [date], our grand opening party will be held on [date].

This letter invites you and your adult family members to visit with us at our new facility on [date] from [—] o'clock to [—] o'clock. The entire staff, including our physicians, will be on hand.

We will serve food and beverages.

Please come and help us celebrate.

Sincerely,

[name]

Templates for Insurance Company-directed External Practice Correspondences

Medicare: Administrative Law Judge Appeal

[date]

RE: [name of patient]
        [patient's Medicare number]
        [patient's control number]
        [date of service]

[inside address]

SUBJECT: Administrative Law Judge Appeal

To the Attention of the Administrative Law Judge:

This is a request for an administrative law judge appeal on a claim that totals [\$—]*.

I have been through carrier review and a fair hearing without success. I received my fair hearing denial [—]† days ago. A copy of my denial is enclosed.

Therefore, I am requesting an "in person" hearing, not an "on-the-record" hearing. The carrier's denial date is [date]. I disagree with the decision of the fair hearing officers because of [—]. To support my request, I have included medical documentation, such as [—]‡. I plan to bring the following witnesses to the appeal: [—].

Please notify me of the time, date, and place of this hearing as soon as possible.

Sincerely,

[name], MD
[physician number]
[UPIN number]

Enclosures

---

*To make this type of appeal, the amount must be more than \$500.
†The fair hearing denial must have been less than 60 days before.
‡List the types of medical documentation that you have included, such as x-rays and laboratory reports.
Send the letter "return receipt requested" and keep the receipt on file.

Medicare: Request for Review of Denied Claim

[date]

RE: [name of patient]
        [patient's Medicare number]
        [patient's control number]

[inside address]

SUBJECT: Medicare Claim Review Request

We are requesting a Medicare claim review because [—].[*]

Please call me at [telephone number] or fax the information to me at [fax number]. I represent [name of practice].

A copy of your remittance statement is enclosed.

Sincerely,

[name]

Enclosure

[*]Give the reasons you are requesting a review of this claim, such as incorrect information was provided.

Medicare: US Department of Health and Human Services Appeals Board

[date]

[inside address]

To the US Department of Health and Human Services Appeals Board:

SUBJECT: Request for Review of Denied Claim

On [date] I received a negative decision from the administrative law judge concerning a claim. The claim is described on the enclosures provided with this letter.

I respectfully request that the appeals board review this claim. I feel confident that the board will reverse the decision after careful review because [—].[*]

The documentation for my belief and supporting medical evidence is enclosed.

Sincerely,

[name], MD

Enclosures

---

[*]Give the reasons you want the claim to be reviewed, such as error in the law, the conclusions of the administrative law judge were not supported, there was an abuse of discretion by the administrative law judge, or there was a policy or procedural issue.

Inadvertent Coding Error

[date]

RE:　　[name of patient]
　　　　[patient's Medicare number]
　　　　[patient's control number]

[inside address]

To [Name of Company]:

An incorrect code for [a/an] [name of procedure]* was submitted on [date].

This [name of procedure] should have been submitted with the diagnosis code of [—] rather than [—].

Please correct this coding error and reprocess this claim for payment.

Sincerely,

[name]

---

*Describe the type of procedure, such as an office visit, consultation, or operation.

Possible Termination of Participation Status

[date]

[inside address]

Dear [name]:

The principals of [name of practice] have met to discuss the group's continued participation with [name of insurance company].

It is the group's consensus that [name of practice] cannot continue to participate with [name of insurance company] under the current reimbursement schedule. To do so will ultimately jeopardize the quality-of-care standards that [name of practice] has established. If [name of insurance company] is interested in entering into negotiations, please contact me at [telephone number]. Otherwise, this letter will serve as official notice of the cancellation of our participation agreement with [name of insurance company] effective [date]. After this date, we will be happy to see [name of insurance company] patients out-of-network.

Please forward the information necessary to terminate the contract so that we may properly advise active beneficiaries (eg, letter of termination to active patients, removal from the Web site, removal from the provider directory, final requests for medical records, etc).

Enclosed with this letter is a report generated by our accounting system listing all open balances and patient names. In advising you of pending termination, we expect prompt resolution of all issues outstanding concerning beneficiaries.

Sincerely,

[name], MD

Directory Error

[date]

[inside address]

To [Name of Insurance Company]:

We have just received our copy of the [city, state] member directory of participating physicians.

Unfortunately, our [—]* was incorrectly listed.

Please correct this error as soon as possible. Our correct [—]* is [—].

Sincerely,

[name]

*State the type of information that was incorrectly listed, such as an address or telephone number.

Lack of Timely Payments

[date]

[inside address]

Dear [name]:

For the [—] month in a row, it has been necessary to make repeated requests for payment to your claims department personnel. This wastes time and causes our staff much aggravation.

Currently, you owe [name of practice] [$—] for claims that we have filed properly and in a timely manner.

The physicians of [name of practice] have come to the decision that, unless we are paid for services rendered to your policyholders within [—] days of our claims submission to you, we will have no choice but to inform our patients that we will no longer honor their coverage with [name of insurance company].

Since [name of insurance company] accounts for [—]% of our annual income, we will also have no choice but to suggest alternative coverage to them.

I will expect your response by [date].

Sincerely,

[name]

Unidentified Payment(s)

[date]

[inside address]

To Whom It May Concern:

We are returning the enclosed [check/checks] totaling [$—], as we are unable to determine if [this patient/these patients] [was/were] seen by the physicians of [name of practice].

It would be extremely beneficial if you would provide us with the treating physician's name and provider number in the future. These are essential to identify a patient's account.

Sincerely,

[name]

Enclosure(s)

Overpayments

[date]

RE: Overpayments

[inside address]

To: [Name of Company]

I am writing to obtain information on how your company handles overpayments to physicians.

Please check the applicable box below, or provide additional information on how your company handles overpayments:

❐   We handle overpayments to physicians by retracting (offsetting) payments on other statements (EOBs) until the overpayment is satisfied.

❐   We send notice to the physician requesting a refund from the physician. We allow ___ days' notice to the physician to satisfy the overpayment.

❐   Other:

_____

_____

_____

After you have completed the survey, please return this letter to me by mail or fax. My fax number is [fax number].

Thank you for your time in helping us better understand your process.

Sincerely,

[name]

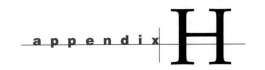

appendix **H**

Templates for Drug Company-directed External Practice Correspondences

Establishing Visit Parameters

[date]

[inside address]

Dear [name]:

On [date], our policy on visits to the practice by pharmaceutical representatives will change. This letter is sent in advance to allow you ample time to adjust your schedule.

Please schedule an appointment with [—] for each of your visits after [same date as above]. The appointments will be approximately [—] minutes each.

We hope this system will be more convenient and will decrease your waiting time in the office.

Sincerely,

[name]

Samples, Instructions, or Literature

[date]

[inside address]

Dear [name]:

In the past we have allowed representatives of pharmaceutical companies to leave samples, instructions, or literature [—].* After [date], we would like to make this process more secure and less labor-intensive for the staff.

After [same date as above], please place your items [—]. Everything will be arranged in an order that should facilitate the process for you.

Thank you for your help in this matter.

Sincerely,

[name]

*Indicate the former location that was used, such as on the table in the conference room.

Sponsor of Charity or Event

[date]

[inside address]

Dear [name]:

This letter is a request to [name of pharmaceutical company] for [$—] to be used to sponsor [name of event or charity].

[Describe event or charity.]*

Please pass this request for [$—] on to the person or department that makes these decisions at [name of pharmaceutical company]. If we count all the practicing physicians who use [name of pharmaceutical company] products, I am only asking for about [—]¢ for every physician.

Thank you in advance for your assistance in this most worthwhile cause.

Sincerely,

[name], MD

Describe the event or charity briefly, along with your involvement with it, and a justification for the request.

Grant for Education in Health Care Careers

[date]

[inside address]

Dear [name]:[*]

Each year or two I encounter very bright young men and women who wish to pursue a medical career (whether it be a nursing career, a pharmaceutical degree, or a doctorate) but lack the funds for education beyond high school. Perhaps they are not eligible for the loans suggested by their school counselors. Or perhaps their parents' income is above the minimum level required for a school loan, but paying back the loan would still prove to be a hardship.

This letter is being sent to seek your assistance in the form of a grant to educate such young people wishing to enter the field of medicine. Does [name of pharmaceutical company] have such a grant program? If so, please send me the details for participation. If not, may I help you start a grant program?

I am grateful for your anticipated response.

Sincerely,

[name], MD

[*]Preferably, this letter should be sent to the CEO or president of the company.

Free Prescription Medication for Needy Patients

[date]

[inside address]

To Whom It May Concern:

Enclosed is the completed form you provided to me to request a [—] [months'/years'] supply of medication for [name of patient].

It is my understanding that the medication will be sent directly to me at my office and I in turn will supply the patient.

Many thanks for this generous and caring effort on the part of [name of pharmaceutical company].

Sincerely,

[name], MD

Thank You

[date]

[inside address]

Dear [name]:

When you faithfully visit us and supply [—],* do you every wonder if we truly appreciate your efforts and those of [name of pharmaceutical company]?

Well, we do! On behalf of the physicians and staff of [name of practice], we want to properly thank you for [—]. Furthermore, we want to thank you for your first-rate character and professional demeanor when you visit us.

Sincerely,

[name]

*Describe the reason for this letter of appreciation, such as lunches provided for the staff.

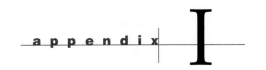

Templates for Physician-directed External Practice Correspondences

Requesting Patient Consultation

[date]

[inside address]

Dear Dr [name]:

I have been treating [name of patient] for [disease/disorder] for [—] [months/years]. [His/Her] [improvement/response to treatment] has been [fair/poor]. I am forwarding the enclosed reports for your review.

If you agree to see [name of patient] for a consultation, I will advise [name of patient] that a member of your office staff will telephone [him/her] to set up a date and time for an appointment.

Please call me at [telephone number] if you have any questions. Thanks for your help.

Sincerely,

[name], MD

Enclosures

Thank You for Patient Referral

[date]

[inside address]

Dear Dr. [name]:

Thank you for referring [name of patient]. I saw [him/her] this morning and believe [he/she] would benefit from [describe treatment]. However, I will reserve final judgment until tests have been completed and the results evaluated.

I will send you a full report by [—]. Meanwhile, I want you to know how much your referrals are appreciated.

Sincerely,

[name], MD

Invitation to Speak

[date]

[inside address]

Dear Dr. [name]:

[Name of organization] has scheduled a [regional/state/national] conference to be held in [city, state] on [date]. The theme of this [—]-day conference is [—].

It is my pleasure to have been asked to invite you to be a guest speaker. The topic we would like addressed is [—]. Your presentation will be scheduled to begin at [—] o'clock on [date] in the [name of room] on the [—] floor of the [—].[*] You should be prepared to conclude your remarks by [—] o'clock.

[Name of organization] [will/will not] pay [—].[†]

If you have any questions, please telephone me at [telephone number]. Please check the box of your choice below and sign your name to accept or decline this invitation. We look forward to having you share your expertise with us.

Sincerely,

[name], MD

❏ I accept   ❏ I decline

_____   _____
Signature   Date

---

[*]Name the facility at which the conference will be held, such as the name of a hotel or other building.
[†]List what will not be paid, such as an honorarium, transportation costs, or food or lodging expenses.

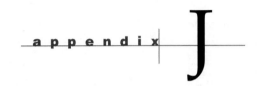

Templates for Home Health Agency-directed External Practice Correspondences

Assuming Care

[date]

RE: [name of patient]
        [patient's address]
        [patient's Social Security number]
        [patient's date of birth]
        [name(s) of patient's insurer(s)]
        [patient's policy number(s)]
        [name of patient's emergency contact]
        [relationship of contact to patient]
        [contact's telephone number]

[inside address]

Dear [name]:*

Please respond to this request [as soon as possible/immediately].

I have been treating [name of patient] for [disease/disorder] for [—] [months/years]. [He/She] requires [—].† [His/Her] [diagnosis/diagnoses] [is/are] [—].

Please contact me as soon as your initial visit has been completed with [weekly/daily] reports of [normal/abnormal] findings thereafter.

Sincerely,

[name], MD

---

*Preferably, this letter should be sent to the intake supervisor of the agency.

†Describe the care the patient requires, such as regular intravenous medication, medical instruction in coping with the illness, or regular monitoring of blood glucose levels.

Fax to the agency and mail the original to ensure receipt, or send the letter "return receipt requested" and keep the receipt on file.

Orders to Be Followed

[date]

RE: [name of patient]
        [patient's address]
        [patient's Social Security number]
        [patient's date of birth]
        [name(s) of patient's insurer(s)]
        [patient's policy number(s)]
        [name of patient's emergency contact]
        [relationship of contact to patient]
        [contact's telephone number]

[inside address]

Dear [name]:[*]

Based on your reports, this patient's [treatment/medication] requires an immediate change.

Please [—].[†]

Please fax me [—][‡] as soon as possible. My fax number is [fax number]. Thank you for your able assistance with this patient.

Sincerely,

[name], MD

---

[*]Preferably, this letter should be sent to the intake supervisor of the agency.

[†]Describe the action to be taken, such as discontinuing, increasing, or decreasing a medication or taking a blood test.

[‡]Describe information that should be faxed, such as laboratory results or the results of the intake supervisor's investigation.

Fax to the agency and mail the original to ensure receipt, or send the letter "return receipt requested" and keep the receipt on file.

Transfer of Patient to Long-term Care

[date]

RE: [name of patient]
   [patient's address]
   [patient's Social Security number]
   [patient's date of birth]
   [name(s) of patient's insurer(s)]
   [patient's policy number(s)]
   [name of patient's emergency contact]
   [relationship of contact to patient]
   [contact's telephone number]

[inside address]

Dear [name]:*

This letter is sent to inform you that [name of patient] now requires long-term skilled nursing care. I have arranged for [him/her] to be transported to [name of nursing home] on [date].

Please suspend your home care services on [date]. Thank you.

Sincerely,

[name], MD

---

*Preferably, this letter should be sent to the director of the agency.

Fax to the agency and mail the original to ensure receipt, or send the letter "return receipt requested" and keep the receipt on file.

Care Complaint

[date]

RE: [name of patient]
         [patient's address]
         [patient's Social Security number]
         [patient's date of birth]
         [name(s) of patient's insurer(s)]
         [patient's policy number(s)]
         [name of patient's emergency contact]
         [relationship of contact to patient]
         [contact's telephone number]

[inside address]

Dear [name]:[*]

[The/A] [—][†] of the above-named patient has reported [—].[‡]

Please investigate this matter further as this is atypical for your organization. Your agency usually provides excellent treatment and care for [name of patient].

Thank you for your assistance, and please contact me with your findings.

Sincerely,

[name], MD

---

[*]Preferably, this letter should be sent to the director of the agency.

[†]Give the relationship of the person who has registered the complaint, such as a daughter, brother, or close friend of the patient.

[‡]Describe the complaint, such as deficient care. Give specifics, such as inadequate bathing of the patient or infrequent visits.

Fax to the agency and mail the original to ensure receipt, or send the letter "return receipt requested" and keep the receipt on file.

Compliments on Care

[date]

[inside address]

Dear [name]:[*]

I want you to know how much I appreciate the care given to all my patients by the staff of [name of home health agency]. Of all the agencies my patients have experienced, yours stands head and shoulders above the rest.

Please convey my gratitude to your staff for the consistently prompt and high-level care that is given to my patients.

Sincerely,

[name], MD

[*]Preferably, this letter should be sent to the director of the agency.

Termination of Care

[date]

RE: [name of patient]
        [patient's address]
        [patient's Social Security number]
        [patient's date of birth]
        [name(s) of patient's insurer(s)]
        [patient's policy number(s)]
        [name of patient's emergency contact]
        [relationship of contact to patient]
        [contact's telephone number]

[inside address]

Dear [name]:*

I have advised the above-named patient and [his/her] family that after [date],† I will no longer be responsible for [name of patient]'s health care. [He/She] has been a consistently noncompliant patient, which gives me no choice but to bow out and allow another physician to try to assist [him/her].

So that your own efforts can be continued, please contact the patient and [his/her] family as soon as possible to ensure that the services of another physician have been secured.

Sincerely,

[name], MD

---

*Preferably, this letter should be sent to the director of the agency.

†This date must be at least 30 days from the date the letter is sent.

Fax to the agency and mail the original to ensure receipt, or send the letter "return receipt requested" and keep the receipt on file.

Request for Care

[date]

RE: [name of patient]
        [patient's address]
        [patient's Social Security number]
        [patient's date of birth]
        [name(s) of patient's insurer(s)]
        [patient's policy number(s)]
        [name of patient's emergency contact]
        [relationship of contact to patient]
        [contact's telephone number]

[inside address]

Dear [name]:*

Please schedule this patient for: †

❑ Physical therapy: for evaluation and treatment
❑ Speech therapy: for evaluation and treatment
❑ Occupational therapy: for evaluation and treatment
❑ Visits with a medical social worker: for evaluation of needs and referral to community resources
❑ Visits with a skilled nurse: to inform patient about the disease process, diet, wound care, and
   medication
❑ Visits with a home health aide: to assist with personal hygiene
❑ Other _____

The frequency and duration of the above will be decided after I have been informed of the results of
your staff evaluation.

Sincerely,

[name], MD

---

*Preferably, this letter should be sent to the director of the agency.
†Check the appropriate box or boxes.
Fax to the agency and mail the original to ensure receipt, or send the letter "return receipt requested" and keep the
receipt on file.

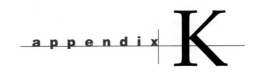
Templates for Other External Practice Correspondences

Termination of Participation in HMO: Letter to Employers

[date]

[inside address]

Dear [name]:*

I regret to inform you that after [date] the physicians of [name of practice] will no longer be participating in [name of HMO].

We realize that this will impact your employees and assure you that we did not come to this decision easily or quickly. For the past [—] years, we have acquiesced to the demands of [name of HMO]. However, we now feel that patient care is being compromised and must withdraw from participation in [name of HMO].

We would like to continue to serve your employee population. Therefore, we have provided you with a list of the insurance plans we will continue to honor.

Sincerely,

[name], MD

Enclosure

*Preferably, this letter should be sent to the CEO of the company.

Nonbinding Letter of Intent for Merger

[date]

[inside address]

Dear Dr. [name]:

SUBJECT: Nonbinding letter of intent for merger

This is a nonbinding letter of intent. The purpose of this letter is to lay the groundwork for a possible merger of your practice with [name of practice].

As the environment of medicine continues to change, physicians across the nation are seeing the need to consolidate through mergers. Some of the main advantages we see in merging with other physicians are:

- Geographic coverage of a larger area for purposes of third-party contracting
- Improved negotiating and financial position through a larger group
- Economics of scale
- Possible coordination and pooling of diagnostic services to achieve efficient utilization

We think it is important that physicians maintain control of their practice entities. For this reason, we are developing a flexible merger model that will allow our practice to merge with other practices to gain the critical mass necessary to survive. This model provides the benefits of a merged entity but also allows each practice to maintain a significant degree of autonomy in daily operations.

The proposal is as follows:

Organizational Divisions

Each group practice that merges with [name of practice] will constitute a division. Each division will remain autonomous in the way it conducts its daily business. Only those issues that are required by law or economics or that the division desires will be determined at the corporate level.

Corporate Level Issues

- Common pension and/or profit-sharing plan
- Standardized nonphysician employee benefits
- Malpractice, life, health, and disability insurance

—Continued

Nonbinding Letter of Intent for Merger—Continued

- From a legal perspective, employment of physician and nonphysician personnel. From an operational perspective, each division will be free to hire and manage their personnel.
- Contractual obligations of the corporation, including debt and provider contracting
- Capital purchases
- Payment of accounts payable
- Billing and collections

Divisional Level Issues

- Physician compensation
- Physician continuing medical education allowances
- Physician vacation and sick and disability leave
- Physician retirement, death, and disability buyouts
- Call schedules and duties
- Hours of operation
- Management of staff (hiring, firing, and discipline)
- Banking

The corporate level personnel will be willing to assume any divisional level issues that you desire. Other than those areas required by law to be placed at the corporate level, you will determine the extent to which these items are shifted from the divisional level to the corporate level.

Revenue Flow

Data entry for services will be entered at the divisional level. Patient statements and insurance claims will be generated at the corporate level. Remittances will be posted and deposited at the divisional level.

Pension Plan

A cross-tested 401(k) and/or profit-sharing plan will be established at the corporate level. The goal of the plan will be to provide maximum flexibility in funding by each physician by division. Each division will determine its funding level in accordance with the plan. Each division will be responsible for funding its contribution for all physicians and nonphysician employees of the division.

Existing Pension Funds

Each division may choose to handle its existing pension funds (subject to approval of legal counsel and compliance with regulatory requirements) according to one of the following:

- By dissolving the plan and allowing each employee to choose between rolling his or her funds into an IRA or into the corporate level plan
- By maintaining funds in an existing plan

Nonbinding Letter of Intent for Merger—Continued

Physician Compensation

Physician compensation formulas will be decided at the divisional level. Once a division has paid its operating expenses, all remaining funds are within the control of the division to compensate physicians. Each division is free to establish its own physician benefit package. Each division is responsible for funding its physician compensation and benefit package.

Accounts Receivable

Each practice is responsible for collecting its own accounts receivable for services generated prior to the merger date. Accounts receivable collection for prior services remains the responsibility of the premerged entity.

Existing Debts

Practices may settle existing premerger debts or carry them into the merged entity. If existing debts are carried into the merged entity, they will be funded from that division's revenue.

Third-Party Payer or Other Liability

Physician employment agreements will contain an indemnification clause whereby physicians will be responsible for any third-party liability assessments, IRS disallowed business expenses, or other similar occurrences.

Hard Assets

Each practice will retain ownership of its hard assets. Under a lease agreement, the hard assets will be leased to the division.

Contracting

Third-party payer contracting will be performed at the corporate level.

Ownership

There are two possible pathways to ownership available. Selection of the most appropriate pathway will be made by the client and legal and/or accounting counsel based on potential tax implications.

Option A. Each physician of each division joins [name of practice] as an employee with a voting seat on the board of directors. The employment relation will continue for a period of [—] years, at which time, if all parties agree, a full merger will occur. The division's current legal entity will remain alive during the [—]-year period to collect the old accounts receivable and hold the division's hard assets.

The main advantage of this option is the ease of exit for the division should the physicians of that division want to extricate themselves from the deal.

Option B. The physicians of each division would merge their practices with [name of practice]. The first level of the merger would entail the division contributing its assets to [name of practice] and the

—Continued

Nonbinding Letter of Intent for Merger—Continued

purchase of a share of [name of practice]'s stock for [$—]. Should a division decide to withdraw, the departing physicians would be entitled to get back the assets they contributed, and their stock would be repurchased for [$—]. Transfer of accounts receivable would be handled as payment of deferred compensation to the departing physicians.

The second level of the merger would entail purchase into the hard assets of the ancillary profit center of the main office. Those physicians wishing to share in the profits of the ancillary department must buy into the department's hard assets. For those physicians who have ownership in these assets, profits of the department may be shared according to the following distribution formula:

- Equally based on ownership percentage
- Prorated based on an indicia, such as gross professional charges
- Based on an arbitrary fixed formula

Profits may not be distributed based on the ordering of tests. Should a physician who has ownership in the ancillary department leave the practice, that physician will be entitled to have his or her share in the ancillary department repurchased according to a predetermined formula.

This is the primary basis of our merger model. If you are interested in the possibility of joining this practice model, please indicate your interest by signing below. Fax [fax number] or mail a copy to me.

Sincerely,

[name], MD

Yes, I am interested in this merger.

_____
Signature

_____
Date

Nondisclosure Agreement

THIS NONDISCLOSURE AGREEMENT was made [date] by [name of first party] and [name of second party].

WHEREAS, [name of second party] is in the business of providing medical services to the general public;

WHEREAS, [name of first party] and [name of second party] wish to explore the possibility of entering into a transaction, the scope of which and form have yet to be determined;

WHEREAS, [name of first party], as part of determining the feasibility of the transaction, desires to review the account books of [name of second party] and, in the course of such review, will acquire valuable knowledge and information concerning the [name of second party] and its accounts and financial operations ("Information"); and

WHEREAS, the Information is confidential and proprietary, and [name of second party] wants to limit access to the Information by individuals employed and/or engaged by [name of first party] and third parties who will have access thereto, and [name of first party] acknowledges and agrees to such limitations as hereinafter set forth.

NOW, THEREFORE, for and in consideration of the sum of [$—], the receipt and sufficiency of which is hereby acknowledged, the parties hereto agree as follows:

The preambles stated above are intended to identify the parties, their intent, and the subject matter hereof. Accordingly, said preambles are incorporated herein as if more fully set forth.

[name of first party] agrees:

Not to communicate any of the Information relating to the [name of second party] to a third party regardless of its physical location, and to use its best efforts to prevent inadvertent disclosure of said Information to any third party;

To limit the distribution of the Information on a need-to-know basis to its employees, accountants, attorneys, and financial advisors, each of whom will sign a written acknowledgment of the terms and provisions of this Agreement, which will be forwarded by [name of first party] to [name of second party];

Not to solicit any party listed on a [name of second party] list provided to [name of first party] for the purpose of offering to the party a service similar to that provided by [name of second party], or which would be competitive with [name of second party];

Not to solicit or employ any of the employees who are currently employed by [name of second party] without the express written consent of [name of second party];

Not to divulge any of the Information, which is confidential in nature, including, without limitation, the financial condition or performance of [name of second party];

Not to establish or cause to be established a business providing medical outpatient services within a [—]-mile radius of the existing [name of second party] business.

In the event [name of first party] should violate any of the provisions of this Agreement, then [name of second party] will be entitled to reasonable attorneys' fees and costs incurred in enforcing [name of second party]'s rights pursuant to this Agreement, and in seeking actual damages in the event of breach.

The obligation of confidence by [name of first party] will not include disclosure of any information, which [name of first party] can document:

—Continued

Nondisclosure Agreement—Continued

Was in the public domain prior to this Agreement or enters the public domain subsequently without breach of this Agreement; or

Was acquired from a third party properly in possession of such Information without any confidential obligation.

The parties agree that each of the covenants and agreements will be deemed severable and separate and the enforceability of any covenant contained herein will not in any manner affect the validity or enforceability of any other covenants set forth herein.

This Agreement will be binding upon and enforceable against the parties hereto, their heirs, successors, personal representatives, and assigns.

Any notice given pursuant to this Agreement will be deemed given when personally delivered against receipt, or sent postage prepaid via the United States mail to the parties at the address below:

Attention: [name of physician or CEO]

_____

Name of first party

_____

Street address

_____

City, state   Zip code

Attention: [name of physician or CEO]

_____

Name of second party

_____

Street address

_____

City, state   Zip code

This Agreement will terminate on [date], at which time [name of first party] will return all copies of the Information provided by [name of second party] and will not retain any copies of the same; provided that the confidentiality provisions of this Agreement will survive such termination and will continue in full force and effect.

The parties agree that this Agreement will be governed and construed in accordance with the laws of [name of state].

This Agreement constitutes the entire agreement between the parties, and may not be amended other than by a written supplemental agreement executed by all parties hereto.

Nondisclosure Agreement—Continued

IN WITNESS WHEREOF, we have hereunto set out hands and seals the day and date first written above.

_____
Name of first party

By:_____
Name of physician or CEO

_____
Date

_____
Name of second party

By:_____
Name of physician or CEO

_____
Date

Nonfulfillment of Obligations by Government Contractor: Letter to Legislator

[date]

[inside address]

Dear [name]:*

SUBJECT: [name of practice]'s contract with [name of HMO]

I am writing to request a meeting on behalf of [name of practice].

On [date], [name of practice] entered into a contractual relationship with [name of HMO]. The purpose of this relationship was the provision of medical services to persons enrolled in [name of HMO]. [Name of practice] has faithfully performed according to contract provisions. Unfortunately, [name of HMO] has not fulfilled its responsibilities according to the agreement.

Since [date], when our problems with [name of HMO] became apparent, [name of practice] has tried to work with [name of HMO] to resolve our differences. The issues outlined below are creating a financial hardship for [name of practice].

- [—]†

Because [name of HMO] is a government contractor, we are seeking intervention from your office.

We are ready to meet with you at your convenience.

Sincerely,

[name], MD

cc: ‡

*Preferably, this letter should be sent to a representative in Congress or a senator.
†List the issues the practice has with the HMO, such as claims processing errors.
‡Send a copy of the letter to the HMO.

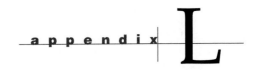
Templates for Correspondences Regarding the Opening of a Practice

Insurance: Requesting Information

[date]

[inside address]

Dear [Name of Insurance Company]:

In [date], I plan to open a medical practice in [city, state]. It is my understanding that your company offers various types of insurance coverage for medical practices.

I am particularly interested in receiving information on [—]*. I would also appreciate learning about other appropriate business indemnifications that I may need and welcome the advice of an experienced broker for my general insurance needs.

Please contact me to arrange a time that is convenient to meet to discuss these vital matters, preferably by June 15, 2004. My telephone number is 909 707-5432, and I am also available by cell phone at 909 685-6459.

Thank you for your assistance. I look forward to your call.
Sincerely,

[name], MD

JD

*Name the type of insurance you want more information about, such as professional liability, disability, property, or worker's compensation.

Insurance: Requesting Participation Status

[date]

[inside address]

RE: Request for participation status

To Whom It May Concern:

My [specialty] practice will open [date] at [street address, city, state, zip code]. My state license number is [—].

I am requesting participating status in [name of insurance company]. Please send me the written requirements and any forms that need to be completed. Please call me at [telephone number] if you have any questions. Or e-mail me at [—] or send your response to [street address, city, state, zip code].

Sincerely,

[name], MD

Seeking an Accountant

[date]

[inside address]

Dear [name]:

SUBJECT: Accounting services

I will be opening a new [specialty] practice in [city, state] in [month] of [year] and am soliciting accounting services.

Please send me information about the services available through your firm, as well as the fees for each.

Thank you for any help you can give me concerning my transition to private practice.

Sincerely,

[name], MD

Seeking an Attorney

[date]

[inside address]

Dear [name]:

SUBJECT: Legal services

On or near [date], I will be opening a medical practice in [city, state] specializing in [specialty].

I need help choosing legal services for my long-term goals. Could you recommend whether [—]* would best suit my needs? Or would you recommend something else entirely?

Please contact me as soon as possible at [telephone number] or e-mail me at [—]. Or send information to [street address, city, state, zip code].

Sincerely,

[name], MD

---

*Give some examples, such as sole practitioner, C-corporation, or S-corporation.

Seeking a Medical Management Consultant

[date]

[inside address]

Dear [name]:

SUBJECT: Medical management consulting services

I am investigating the possibility of employing a medical management consultant to assist with the opening of a new practice specializing in [specialty]. The practice will be located in [city, state] and my anticipated opening date is [date].

I am especially interested in [—].*

Please let me know if you or others in your firm can assist in [this area/these areas]. Please send me information about your firm's credentials and the duration of your medical consulting experience.

Also, please send me a list of at least [number] practicing physicians who are clients of yours, along with their addresses and/or telephone numbers.

Sincerely,

[name], MD

---

*Give some examples of the area(s) you are interested in, such as computer selection, job descriptions, marketing, establishing fees, coding, setting wage and salary scales, and/or recruiting staff.

Obtaining a State Medical License

[date]

[inside address]

RE: Obtaining a [—]* medical license

To Whom It May Concern:

Please send me the necessary information and requirements for obtaining a medical license in the state of [—].*

I received my medical degree from [medical school] in [year] and completed my residency training at [—] in [year].

Please send your transmittal to me at [street address, city, state, zip code]. Or you can fax the information to me at [fax number].

Sincerely,

[name], MD

*Name the state, such as Florida.

Obtaining a City or County Business License

[date]

[inside address]

SUBJECT: Obtaining a [city/county] business license

Dear [city/county] Business License Office

I plan to open a medical practice in [city/county] in [month, year]. However, I am unfamiliar with the business license procedures to be followed in [city/county]. I would appreciate receiving the necessary information concerning meeting the legal requirements for business licensing. Please send the information to me at [street/city/state/zip] so that I can meet the requirements.

Sincerely,

[name], MD

Obtaining a Drug Enforcement Administration (DEA) Certificate

[date]

[inside address]

SUBJECT: Obtaining a Drug Enforcement Administration (DEA) Certificate

On [date] I plan to begin practicing medicine at [street address, city, state, zip code]. This letter is my request for a DEA certificate application. Also, please include literature that contains the appropriate rules and regulations.

The requested data may be sent to me at the above address.

Sincerely,

[name], MD

Seeking Hospital Privileges

[date]

[inside address]

Dear [name]:[*]

After [date], I will be practicing medicine full-time in [city, state]. It is my intention to admit patients to [name of hospital].

Please send me a summary of your medical staff bylaws, along with an application for active privileges. If you can provide me with a roster of the active physicians on your staff, this would also be appreciated. Thank you.

Sincerely,

[name], MD

[*]Preferably, this letter should be sent to the administrator or CEO of the hospital.

Requesting Subscriptions From a Central Source

[date]

[inside address]

To Whom It May Concern:

It is my understanding that, rather than dealing with each publisher individually, your firm can provide me with all the subscriptions I need for my new office-based practice. I would like delivery to start as of [date].

I am interested in receiving the following on a weekly or monthly basis, according to the individual publisher's schedules: [—].[*]

Please advise me of the annual rates for these periodicals.

Sincerely,

[name], MD

---

[*]List the names of the magazines, newspapers, and journals.

Requesting Bids for Copiers

[date]

[inside address]

Dear ABC Copier Company:

Please send us pricing for copier-related supplies and services for the opening of a medical practice. The practice will be in [city, state], where the equipment will be delivered, used, and serviced. We will need this equipment no earlier than [date] and no later than [date].

Please direct any questions about this matter to [name]. [He/She] is also the person to whom you should send your bid and pricing information within [—] [days/weeks] of receipt of this letter.

Please include in the bid how much it will cost on a yearly basis to own and operate the equipment.

We [will/will not]* be trading in equipment.

The equipment we require [—].†

Please indicate any known delays associated with delivery or receipt of the equipment.

Concerning shipping, invoices, and payments, [—].‡

Please provide a service agreement that includes information on on-site repairs and servicing during normal business hours. We would prefer service within [—] business days of the service call. Are [—]§ included in the service agreement?

Also, please send the names, addresses, and telephone numbers of at least [—] local clients who have purchased similar supplies and services from you.

Sincerely,

[name], MD

---

*If you will be trading in equipment, mention the type and model number, when the equipment was purchased, how much it was used (how many copies were made), and the company that serviced it. Ask for the value of the trade-in equipment in writing.

†Describe the necessary equipment and basic features, such as copies a month; collating, speed, stapling, single- or double-sided copy, reducing or enlarging, and/or mechanical- or manual-feed capability; type and size of paper, and/or ease of replenishing paper, resolving paper jams, or selecting settings. Mention if space is limited (give dimensions).

‡Describe how you want matters handled, such as shipping documents or invoices accepted as payment requests and/or payment authorized and sent upon acceptance of supplies.

§Describe what you want included in the service agreement, such as toner or drum replacement.

Requesting Proposals for Computer Hardware or Software

[date]

[inside address]

Dear Sales Manager:

We are requesting pricing for [—].[*]

Features that we deem to be essential include [—].[†]

Training and support are very important to us. We are located in [city, state]. We are also very price conscious and are considering at least [—] other systems.

We would like installation and training to be completed by [date].

Please reply as soon as possible. Your proposal should identify specific equipment and applications.

Sincerely,

[name], MD

[*]Describe the type of hardware or software for which you are requesting pricing.
[†]Describe essential features, such as keeping track of appointments, billing, claims, and/or office expenses.

Real Estate: Renting or Buying Office Space

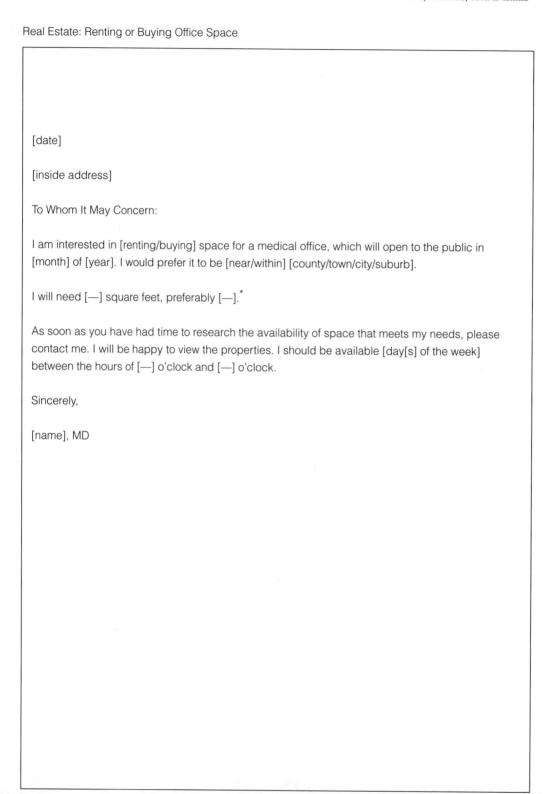

[date]

[inside address]

To Whom It May Concern:

I am interested in [renting/buying] space for a medical office, which will open to the public in [month] of [year]. I would prefer it to be [near/within] [county/town/city/suburb].

I will need [—] square feet, preferably [—].*

As soon as you have had time to research the availability of space that meets my needs, please contact me. I will be happy to view the properties. I should be available [day[s] of the week] between the hours of [—] o'clock and [—] o'clock.

Sincerely,

[name], MD

*State what you would prefer, such as office space close to elevators or on the ground floor.

Real Estate: Rental Agreement Modification

[date]

[inside address]

Dear [name]:

Thank you for your proposal dated [date]. I am prepared to proceed provided we can agree to the following modifications: [—].[*]

Your proposal and this letter should not be construed as a legally binding offer to lease the space. If the above is agreeable, please forward a lease to me for review. Feel free to call me to discuss this proposal.

When can we meet to finalize the agreement? I am available [date] or [date].

Sincerely,

[name], MD

[*]List the proposed modifications to the agreement, such as rent escalation rate, availability of parking spaces, restriction on other physicians within the development area, relocation of the bathrooms, and/or renewal policy.

Templates for Correspondences Regarding the Closing of a Practice

Notifying Employees

[date]

[inside address]

Dear [name]:

In [—][weeks/months], [I/we] plan to close [my/our] medical practice. The last day open will be [date]. You have been a member of a very capable and supportive team, for which [I/we] thank you.

It is [my/our] hope that you will remain through the last day of operation. However, [I/we] realize that you must think of your next opportunity for employment and take advantage of any opening when it occurs. Those who remain employed at [name of practice] until the final day will receive a bonus check equivalent to [—] [weeks'/months'] salary. [I/We] hope you will be among those remaining until the last day.

You may expect a favorable reference for your excellent work and loyalty.

On [date], we will meet from [—] o'clock to [—] o'clock to resolve any questions you might have about this process. We will discuss such topics as [—].[*] Please prepare your questions in advance so that our time may be used productively.

The last day to schedule patients for appointments will be [date].

Thank you for everything you have done to make [my/our] [life/lives] and that of our patients more rewarding.

Sincerely,

[name], MD

[*]List the topics that will be discussed, such as the pension plan or earned but unpaid or unused vacation time.

Notifying Patients

[date]

[inside address]

Dear [name]:

After [date], I will no longer be able to care for your medical needs. I plan to [—].*

Assisting you with your medical care has made my life satisfying and productive. I hope my family and hobbies will help fill any void.

Enclosed is an authorization for the release of your medical records. Please complete the [form/forms], sign [it/them], and return [it/them] to the office. I can then send your records to any physician you select.

The following local physicians have indicated to me that they are willing to accept new patients: [—].†

I offer this list only for your convenience. You need not select from this list. Please consider other factors, such as your medical insurance, when selecting another physician.

I hope this notice will give you ample time to attend to prescription refills, transfer of records, and, for those who wish, a final visit with me!

Sincerely,

[name], MD

*Explain what your plans are, such as to retire or move out of state.
†List a few physicians, along with the name of their practice, practice address, and office telephone number.

Notifying Hospitals

[date]

[inside address]

RE: Voluntary withdrawal of admitting privileges

Dear [name]:[*]

On [date] I plan to retire from medical practice. It is with mixed emotions that I request that my [specialty] admitting privileges be withdrawn.

Please ensure that the hospital records reflect that this is a voluntary withdrawal of privileges. It is my pleasure to have been able to serve my patients at [name of hospital].

Sincerely,

[name], MD

[*]Preferably, this letter should be sent to the administrator of the hospital.

Notifying Colleagues

[date]

[inside address]

Dear Dr [name]:*

The time has come! [Date] will be my last day of practice.

It has been my distinct pleasure to have known you and worked with you throughout the years. Keep up the good work.

Sincerely,

[name], MD

---

*Or, if the physician is also a personal friend, address him or her by first name.

Notifying Insurance Companies

[date]

[inside address]

To [Name of Insurance Company]

RE: Closing of medical practice

On [date] I plan to cease practicing. You will continue to receive insurance claim forms for [—] [weeks/months] afterwards as we follow up on unpaid, pending, and unfiled claims. However, there will be no dates of service after [date as above]. This information is sent for your protection and mine.

After [date] any correspondence from you, including remittances, should be sent to [street address, city, state, zip code].

Thank you for your attention to this matter.

Sincerely,

[name], MD

Send the letter "return receipt requested" and keep the receipt on file.

Notifying Lessor

[date]

[inside address]

Dear [name]:

SUBJECT: Notice of Intent to Vacate Rental Office Space

[I/we] plan to vacate the rental space at [street address, city, state] on [date].

According to the lease, [I/We] must provide [—] days' notice, which [I/we] [am/are] [providing at this time/regretfully cannot provide].[*]

The final rent check will be sent to you as usual on [date]. If there are any contingencies to be settled, please contact [name].

Sincerely,

[name], MD

[*]If you have not provided sufficient notice, explain what arrangements will be made to rectify he matter.
Send the letter "return receipt requested" and keep the receipt on file.

Notifying Utilities

[date]

Re: Name of Account
         Account Number
         Street Address
         City, State, Zip Code

[inside address]

SUBJECT: Discontinuation of [—]* service as of [date]

[I/We] plan to vacate the office space at [street address, city, state] on [date].

Please arrange for service to be disconnected by [date].

The final statement for service may be sent to [street address, city, state, zip code]. Thank you for your assistance.

Sincerely,

[name], MD

*State the type of service that will be discontinued, such as telephone, gas, or electricity.
Send the letter "return receipt requested" and keep the receipt on file.

Notifying Professional Liability Insurer

[date]

Re: Termination of professional liability insurance [policy number]

[inside address]

Dear [Name of Company]:

My last day of active medical practice will be [date]. Please end my professional liability insurance at [—] o'clock on the same date.

If there is an unearned premium to be refunded to me, please send it to [street address, city, state, zip code].

Please contact me immediately concerning termination of this insurance and the possibility of obtaining other types of coverage. [—]*

Sincerely,

[name], MD

---

*If you have "occurrence" coverage, "tail" coverage may not be necessary. However, if you have a "claims made" policy, you must purchase tail coverage or obtain "nose" coverage.

Send the letter "return receipt requested" and keep the receipt on file.

Notifying Other Insurers

[date]

Re: Termination of insurance coverage [policy number]

[inside address]

Dear [Name of Agent/Company]:

After [date] I will no longer require your insurance coverage as I am closing my medical practice.

Please contact me before [date] so that we can tie up all loose ends concerning this matter.

Sincerely,

[name], MD

Send the letter "return receipt requested" and keep the receipt on file.

Notifying the Drug Enforcement Administration (DEA)

[date]

[inside address]

To Whom It May Concern:

Subject: Voluntary surrendering of DEA privileges [DEA number]

I would like to surrender my DEA privileges as I plan to close my office and stop practicing medicine on [date].

Please provide me with instructions for the disposal of narcotics and other classified drugs in my possession. Thank you for your assistance.

Sincerely,

[name], MD

Send the letter "return receipt requested" and keep the receipt on file.

Notifying Specialty Board

[date]

[inside address]

Dear [Name of Entity]:

After [date] I will no longer practice medicine.

Accordingly, please move my name from active to inactive status.

Sincerely,

[name], MD

Notifying Medical Societies

[date]

[inside address]

Dear [name]:

I plan to stop practicing medicine on [date]. Please place my records with the society into inactive status after this time.

Please send any future correspondence to me to [street address, city, state, zip code].

It has been my pleasure to have been a member of [name of society].

Sincerely,

[name], MD

Records: Storage Inquiry

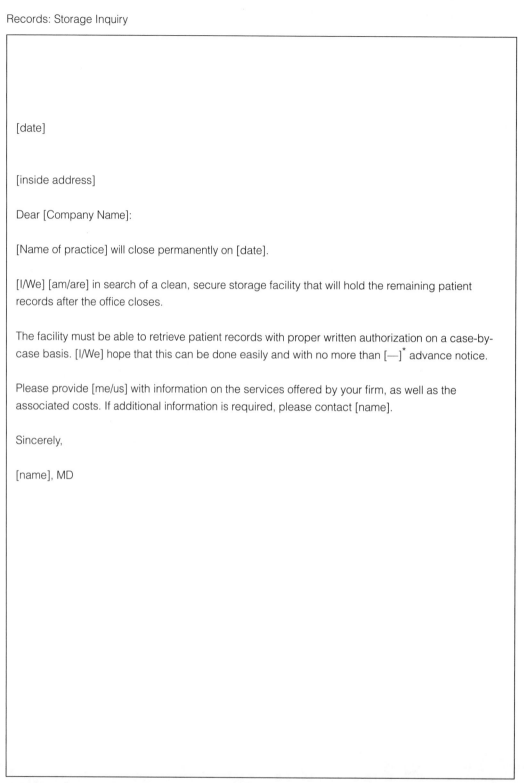

[date]

[inside address]

Dear [Company Name]:

[Name of practice] will close permanently on [date].

[I/We] [am/are] in search of a clean, secure storage facility that will hold the remaining patient records after the office closes.

The facility must be able to retrieve patient records with proper written authorization on a case-by-case basis. [I/We] hope that this can be done easily and with no more than [—]* advance notice.

Please provide [me/us] with information on the services offered by your firm, as well as the associated costs. If additional information is required, please contact [name].

Sincerely,

[name], MD

*State how much advance notice you think is reasonable, such as 24 hours.

Records: Microfilm Inquiry

[date]

[inside address]

Dear [Name of Company]:

[My/Our] medical practice office will close permanently on [date] and [I/we] would like information about your microfilm services, including storage and retrieval.

Please provide [me/us] with information regarding the cost of microfilming, storing, and retrieving medical records. The records are, on average, [—] by [—]* and there are approximately [—] of them.

Easy retrieval with proper authorization is very important. If additional information is required, please contact [name] at [telephone number]. Thank you for any help you can give concerning this matter.

Sincerely,

[name], MD

*State the average size of the pages that are to be microfilmed, such as 8.5" x 11".

Records: Advisory to Patients on Disposition of Records

[date]

[inside address]

Dear [name]:

Medical records from [name of practice] that were not transferred to another physician are now in storage. [—] is the name of the storage facility. It is located at [street address, city, state, zip code].

To retrieve your medical records, please telephone [name of facility] at least [—] hours in advance of pickup. The telephone number of the facility is [telephone number].

Sincerely,

[name], MD

It is also advisable to place a notice in local newspapers.

Uncollected Accounts: Billing Company or Collection Agency Inquiry

[date]

[inside address]

To [Name of Company]:

[I/We] closed [name of practice] on [date] and have more than [—] uncollected accounts totaling approximately [$—].

If your firm is interested in pursuing the collection of these funds, please contact [name].

Sincerely,

[name], MD

Uncollected Accounts: Patient Advisory

[date]

[inside address]

Dear [name]:

[Name of billing company/collection agency] has been authorized to collect all funds owed to [name of practice].

Sincerely,

[name], MD

Terminating Subscriptions From a Central Source

[date]

RE: Name of Practice
        Account Number
        Street Address
        City/State/Zip Code

[inside address]

Dear [Name of Company]:

After [date], please cancel the subscriptions to the following publications: [—].*

Refund the unused portion of the payments to [name of practice]. Please contact [name] if you have further questions.

Sincerely,

[name], MD

*List the names of the magazines, newspapers, or journals.

Terminating Services

[date]

RE: Name of Practice
        Account Number
        Street Address
        City/State/Zip Code

[inside address]

To Whom It May Concern:

[Name of practice] will close permanently on [date] and will no longer require regular [—]* service after this date.

The final pickup should take place, as scheduled, on [date]. Thank you for your past service.

Sincerely,

[name]

*State the type of services you are terminating, such as linen service or the disposal of hazardous materials.

Cowan J. *Techniques for Communicators*. Chicago, Ill: Lawrence Ragan Communications, Inc.

Cramer P, Smith D. *How to Create High-Impact Letters and Memos*. Boulder, Colo: CareerTrack Publications; 1994.

Damsey J. *Handbook of Physician Office Letters*. Chicago, Ill: AMA Press; 2000.

Kinderman KL. *Medicolegal Forms With Legal Analysis: Documenting Issues in the Patient-Physician Relationship*. Chicago, Ill: American Medical Association; 1999.

Lauchman R. *Plain Style: Techiniques for Simple, Concise, Emphatic Business Writing*. New York, NY: Amacom; 1993.

Strunk W, White EB, Angell R. *Elements of Style*. 4th ed. New York, NY: Pearson Higher Education; 2000.

Whitman D. *The Road to Readability: Basics of Writing and Editing*. Chicago, Ill: Lawrence Ragan Communications, Inc; 1993.

INDEX

A

Abbreviations, for forms of address, titles, and academic degrees, 90–91

Academic degrees, abbreviations for, 90–91

Accountants, template for seeking, 212

Active verbs, 14–15

Addresses
abbreviations for forms of, 90–91
delivery, 35–38
return, 38–39

Addressing
exceptional, 39
guidelines for, 39t
occupant, 39
simplified, 39

Adjustments, credit, 59–60

Administrative law judge appeal, template for, 170

Advance deposit account, 43

Ancillary service endorsements, 39–40

Announcements
letters for, 55
memorandums for, 67

Apology, letters of, 56–57

Appointment reminders, template for, 158

Assuming care, template for, 192

Attorneys, template for seeking, 213

Automation-compatible mail, 43

B

Balloon rate, 43

Benefits, overutilization of, template for, 136

Billing companies, template for finding, 241

Block formats, for professional letters, 29–30

Boards, specialty, template for notifying practice closings to, 236

Bottom margins, for professional letters, 28

Bulk mail, 43

Bulk mail center (BMC), 43

Business letters. *See* Professional letters

Business mail entry unit (BMEU), 43

C

Care, templates for home health agency-directed
assuming, 192
for complaints, 195
for compliments, 196
orders to be followed, 193
for requests for, 198
for termination of, 197
transfer of patient to long-term, 194

Carrier route presort mail, 43

City licenses, obtaining, template for, 216

Clichés, avoiding, 13

Closings, for professional letters, 22. *See also* Practice closings

Clustering, 9, 10f

COBRA, templates for
death of employee, 130
divorce or legal separation, 131
employees with Medicare, 132

Coding errors, inadvertent, template for, 173

Collection agencies, template for finding, 241

Collection letters, 60–61, 161–164

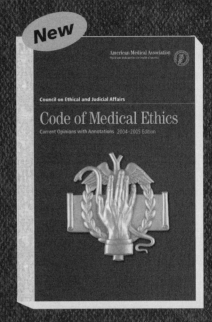

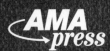

CD-ROM INSTALLATION INSTRUCTIONS

The *Handbook of Medical Office Communications: Effective Letters, Memos, and E-mails* CD-ROM (located at the back of this book) is a cross-platform CD-ROM that will run on both Windows-based and Macintosh PCs. To install the CD-ROM, follow these steps:

Windows Users

1. Insert the CD into your CD-ROM drive.
2. If AutoPlay is enabled, the CD will open automatically to reveal the letter files.
3. Double click any of the files that appear in the CD window to access the files on the CD-ROM.

If Autoplay is *not* enabled and the CD-ROM does not open automatically, follow these steps:

1. Select the DESKREF CD-ROM icon (or the icon that designates your CD drive) that appears on your desktop or in the My Computer window (select Start > My Computer) and double click to display its contents. You should see the letter files.
2. Double click any of the files that appear in the CD window to access the files on the CD-ROM.

Macintosh Users

1. Insert the CD into your CD-ROM drive.
2. Double click the DESKREF CD-ROM icon that appears on your desktop to open the CD-ROM and display its contents. You should see the letter files.
3. Double click any of the files that appear in the CD window to access the files on the CD-ROM.

Minimum System Requirements

Windows
- CD-ROM drive
- Pentium-class processor
- Microsoft Windows
- 64 MB RAM
- Microsoft Word 97/98 or later

Macintosh
- CD-ROM drive
- PowerPC processor
- Apple Mac OS 9.0 or later
- 64 MB RAM
- Microsoft Word 98 or later